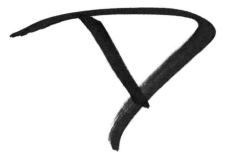

Goddess Power

Every girl is a goddess! When you access your goddess power, you can make your life exactly as you want it to be. Yes, sometimes people may do things that hurt you; yes, sometimes disappointments or accidents happen.

I asked the Goddess why we go through hard times, and this is what she said:

> "Problems and difficulties are not to be feared but to be faced—head-on. They are gifts that initiate you into a different person, a wiser person, a more discerning person. They give you greater empathy, greater compassion, and deeper love. It is not the problem or difficulty that undermines you, but the way that you tackle it."

So use your goddess power and be a GIRL—Goddess In Real Life! Remarkable things will happen when you begin to delve into your divine beauty and listen to the inner voice of the Goddess.

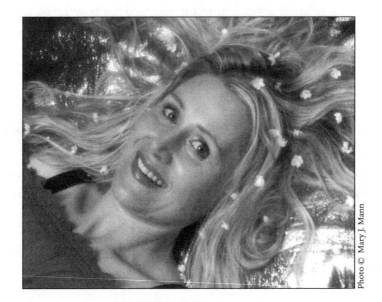

Photo © Mary J. Mann

About the Author

Catherine Wishart has been practicing goddess magic and metaphysics for twenty years. She graduated from the prestigious Aveda Horst Education Center with honors and has worked as a skin-care specialist. She teaches goddess workshops in the United States, New Zealand, and Australia. Currently, Catherine resides in New Mexico with her family. Check out her website, www.talktoyourangels.com, for information about classes and personal readings.

TEEN GODDESS

How to
**LOOK, LOVE
& LIVE**
like a
GODDESS

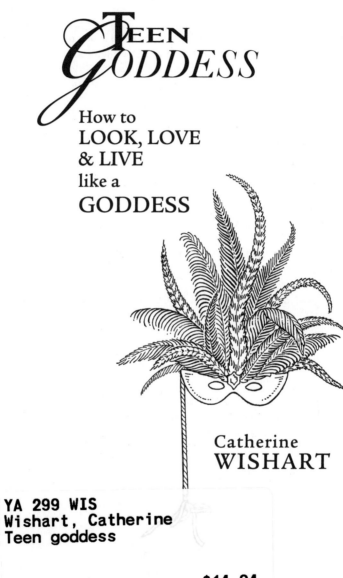

Catherine
WISHART

2003
Llewellyn Publications
St. Paul, Minnesota 55164-0383, U.S.A.

FIRST EDITION
First Printing, 2003

Book design and editing by Rebecca Zins
Cover design by Gavin Dayton Duffy
Cover photo by Ann Brown/Superstock ©2002
Mask illustration © Kate Thomssen

Library of Congress Cataloging-in-Publication Data
Wishart, Catherine, 1965-
    Teen goddess : how to look, love & live like a goddess / Catherine Wishart.—1st ed.
        p. cm.
    ISBN 0-7387-0392-3
    1. Magic. 2. Goddesses—Miscellanea. 3. Teenage girls—Miscellanea. 4. Beauty, Personal—Miscellanea. 5. Goddess religion. 6. Teenage girls—Religious life. I. Title.

BF1623.G63W57 2003
299–dc21   2003040112

Llewellyn Worldwide does not participate in, endorse, or have any authority or responsibility concerning private business transactions between our authors and the public.

All mail addressed to the author is forwarded but the publisher cannot, unless specifically instructed by the author, give out an address or phone number.

Any Internet references contained in this work are current at publication time, but the publisher cannot guarantee that a specific location will continue to be maintained. Please refer to the publisher's website for links to authors' websites and other sources.

Llewellyn Publications
A Division of Llewellyn Worldwide, Ltd.
P.O. Box 64383, Dept. 0-7387-0392-3
St. Paul, MN 55164-0383, U.S.A.
www.llewellyn.com

Printed in the United States of America

For Dad

You've got to get up every morning,
look in the mirror, and say to yourself,
"Today is going to be the best day of my life!"
—RON WISHART (1924–)

I love you!

Acknowledgments

Special thanks to:

My dear husband Stephen, my *Anam Cara*, thank you for all the love and devotion you give me and for holding my hand on our journey together. Thanks for being you, honey. You are the best.

Logan and Kylan, our two beautiful boys. You teach me so much about magic every day. I just love being your mum.

Oz Anderson, for your friendship, love, and support, not to mention all the wonderful magical journeys we have undertaken together.

Elena Avila, for being such a wonderful teacher and showing me how to contain and use my own goddess power.

Misha Crosbie and Jessica Fleming, my two dear fairy godmothers, who have midwived me through many turning points in my life.

Aaron Hendren, for all our writing conversations.

Maya Sutton, for your dear friendship and your unwavering belief in my work.

Kaila Yorke, for your constant and loyal friendship.

How lucky I am to have such blessed friends.

Thanks also to Doreen Virtue and Bronny Daniels, for your generosity of spirit. You truly walk your talk.

Many thanks to the dream team at Llewellyn—Becky, Megan, Jill, Heather, Lisa, Gavin, and Meghan—whose talent and expertise birthed this book in the most beautiful way possible.

And special thanks to Leslie Kenton, who was my unseen mentor when I was a teenager. Through your beauty writings, I was inspired to find my path.

Contents

How to use this book   *xi*

Writing this book . . .   *xiii*

SECTION ONE: THE BASICS

So what is a goddess anyway?   3

Magic 101   21

Awakening your inner goddess   37

Gifts of the inner goddess   55

Conjuring your destiny   77

SECTION TWO: THE GODDESSES

The goddess glamours   99

Inanna: goddess of weighty matters   103

Scathach: punk rock warrior goddess   119

Queen Boadicea: the avenging goddess   139

Bridget: goddess of inspiration and healing   157

Sarasvati: goddess of schoolwork, music, and sensuality   173

Huesuda: the gothic goddess   189

Kuan Yin: goddess of compassion and forgiveness   209

Freya: the air goddess   227

Mahuika: the fire goddess   243

Oshun: the water goddess   267

Mary: the moon goddess   283

Grania: the sun goddess   303

Gaia: the earth goddess   325

La Llorona: the starving goddess   343

Aphrodite: the beauty goddess   361

Conclusion   *379*

Further reading   *385*

Index   *389*

How to use this book

This book is a workbook—I can provide you with the information but, in order for you to access your goddess power, you need to practice it. Use this information and make it your own. Write in the margins, underline what you like, cross out what you don't. Make this *your* goddess book.

Your goddess power is unique to you; you are the only goddess like you on the whole planet—pretty awesome, huh? So let's get going. All you need to begin is an open mind and an open heart. I encourage you to get a special journal—your goddess diary—to take notes and keep track of your goddess training. Think of it as your goddess logbook.

This book is divided into two sections: the basics and the goddesses. Please read the basics first as they will lay the foundation for the goddess chapters. You can read each goddess chapter in any order you wish. Just choose a goddess that seems kind of fun to you. My suggestion is to work with each goddess for a week before moving on to the next. At the end of the book, you will know how to throw a glamour for fifteen different goddesses. But don't stop there. Find another goddess to work with and make up your own glamours. I'd love to hear about what you do—so write me if you get a chance, okay?

Whenever you see a Goddess Workout header, there's something for you to try. These workouts will get you thinking and provide tasks for you to do—just like Aphrodite made Psyche complete certain tasks to initiate her into the realm of her own goddess power, so I will provide certain challenges for you. These tasks are designed to bring you closer to your understanding of the Goddess. Consider them soul stretches. Read the workout through once before doing it because sometimes I will ask you to close your eyes and visualize certain things. Grab a pen as you read and get ready to go. . . .

My wish for this book is simple. I hope it will teach you how to make your life more magical.

May the Goddess love you, bless you, and guide you, now and forever!

Catherine

Writing this book . . .

As I wrote this book, lots of amazing things happened. For each chapter I worked on, the goddess I was writing about would show me things in my dreams or tell me things as I was writing. Very often I felt like a scribe, writing down what I could hear the goddess saying. Plus the goddesses would tell me stuff about themselves as I was writing their stories. Sometimes they would want to add things or change the way they have been perceived in recent times.

At each chapter, it seemed like I was working on that particular message in my own life. For example, Kuan Yin beckoned me to stretch my heart with compassion and forgive those I held a grudge against, and Oshun challenged me to take responsibility for managing my moods all the time! Mary helped me understand the sacred relationship between mothers and children. I cried as I wrote her story because I could feel her intense pain at losing her son. For each chapter, the goddesses made me do the work. My life is richer for it. And I know the goddesses will be there for you as you read each chapter, nudging you forward to do the work, too.

SECTION ONE

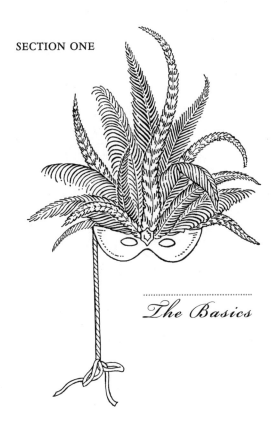

The Basics

So What Is a Goddess Anyway?

You Are a Goddess

You are a goddess. Did you know that? All the power, strength, and magic that was available to the ancient goddesses is available to you today. You carry the divinity, beauty, and wisdom of the ancient goddesses within you. You don't have to do anything to earn it. It is already there. Throughout this book I will show you how to access your goddess power and how to use it to make your life exactly as you would like it to be.

You can use your goddess power to help you with any area of your life, from getting a boyfriend to losing weight, passing exams, and strengthening your confidence. As you learn how to tune into your divine nature, you will learn to listen to your inner voice, the voice of Spirit talking to you, and remarkable things will begin to happen. You will notice that coincidences and synchronicities will take place on a regular basis. You will effortlessly become more attractive and you will feel more confident about your ability to make decisions. Most importantly, you will feel confident about yourself.

What Is a Goddess?

Whenever I talk about goddesses, my friend Liarne always asks, "What is a goddess?" What exactly do I mean when I use the word goddess? Am I referring to the goddesses from ancient myths who had strange and magical powers? Do I mean that women are goddesses? Or am I talking about the goddesses whom people used to worship and continue to do so in some religions around the world? Yes! Yes, and yes!

But before I tell you what *I* think a goddess is, why don't you tell me what *you* think a goddess is?

Goddess Workout

Take a minute now. Take a deep breath and close your eyes. What words or images spring to mind when you think of a goddess? Do you ever think about the concept of a goddess? What does the word "goddess" mean to you?

Write or draw your answers here:

A goddess, to me, is . . .

Who are some goddesses you already know (real or imagined)?

Are there any women you would consider goddesses? Who? And why?

Perhaps as you read this book your understanding of what a goddess is will change. When you get to the end, come back to those questions you've just answered and compare your thoughts.

My dictionary defines a goddess as:

- A female god or deity

- A greatly adored woman

- A woman of great beauty

To me a goddess is all these things, and much more. When I talk about the Goddess I am referring to the divine feminine. I believe we are all manifestations of the divine. Therefore, if you are a female, you are a *divine* female and thus a goddess. Whenever I refer to the Goddess, as opposed to a specific goddess with a name, I am talking about the divine feminine—the one whom ancient peoples worshipped as the mother of all.

When I think of the Goddess, I see a wise and beautiful woman who looks like a fairy queen with big, luminescent wings and a long, flowing gown. She is like my guardian angel, someone who is always there, guiding me every second of the day. How the Goddess appears to you may be completely different. You may see a divine mother, a celestial being, or a strong, muscled warrior. Goddesses, like women, appear in many different forms with many different attributes.

Throughout this book you will get to know some specific goddesses from different cultures. You will discover what their strengths were and how they can help you today. You will also learn what challenges they faced, how they overcame them, and how you can overcome similar challenges in your own life. As you learn about the different goddesses, you may find a patron goddess. You may feel drawn to work with a particular goddess, or one may choose to take you under her wing. Ever since I was twenty-one, Aphrodite, the Greek goddess of love, has been my patron goddess. She is the goddess I work with on a daily basis. At various times of my life, different goddesses have aided me. Grania, the Celtic sun goddess, is who I am working with as I write now. As you will see, there are many different goddesses whom people have honored since time began.

The Goddess Through the Ages

Nearly all ancient cultures worshipped the Goddess in one form or another. During the Paleolithic era, which took place from 50,000 B.C.E. (before common era) to 8000 B.C.E., people revered the Goddess as the mother of all. These people painted the Goddess in the caves where they lived and made sculptures to honor her over 35,000 years ago. Hundreds of goddess figurines dating back to that era have been found across Europe, from as far afield as the Pyrenees Mountains in France all the way to the plains of Siberia. Most of these statues are small, naked, and pregnant, showing the Goddess in her life-giving aspect.

The Goddess, as the Earth, was honored for her fertility. She produced life from her body—plentiful crops for people to eat, rain and water in springs and rivers. The livelihood of the tribes depended on her abundance. Many of the goddess statues were painted with red ochre to symbolize the blood of life that sustains us all.

Women in Paleolithic times were honored, too, for their ability to give birth. Children took their mother's names rather than their father's, and in that way no child was illegitimate. Women, like the Earth, could sustain life from their bodies, feeding their babes from the milk that flowed from their breasts, just as the Earth Mother fed her children—humans, plants, and animals—from the foods and waters that flowed from her body.

At that point in time, giving birth was a mystery. As far as we know, the ancient Stone Age people had no concept that men even contributed to the birth of a child. Birth was one of the mysteries of womanhood, as was menstruation. Women's menstrual cycles followed a twenty-eight-day cycle, just as the moon did. In those days, people followed a lunar calendar rather than a solar one, so there were thirteen months in the year instead of our twelve. Women, too, had thirteen periods each year. This close association of women with the cycles of nature was obvious and revered. Women were thought to contain mystical powers that enabled them to give birth.

The tribes lived inside caves, making their homes near the entrance. Deeper into the caves they would paint beautiful pictures of the Goddess on the dark walls using bright reds, dusty yellows, and rich chocolatey browns. Outside their front doors, at the mouth of the cave, they would place statues of the Goddess. In their hands or their carry packs, where they kept their tools, they would carry small goddess statues.

These statues had large, pendulous breasts, ample hips, lush thighs, and a round, pregnant belly, representing the Goddess giving birth to everything on Earth from her bountiful body. Like the Earth, her body was round, rolling, and rich. She is faceless, indicating that she is the sacred female embodiment of all. Most of these figurines had feet that pointed downward in an arrowlike shape, probably to make it easier to stick them in the ground outside the homes. The statues were carved either from stone or bone.

One of the most famous statues from that time is the goddess of Willendorf, who was found in 1908 near Willendorf in Austria. She is over 30,000 years old and is one of the oldest pieces of artwork found on the planet. She was found among some tools from that era and was carved out of limestone. Most commonly she is known as the Venus of Willendorf; however, Venus was a goddess who did not appear until later in the history of humankind.

Why did ancient people carve images of the Goddess? Well, shamans have long believed the spirit world is close at hand, superimposed over the physical world we see rather than miles away in some far-off land. Think of it in computer graphic terms. Let's say you are working on an image with several layers. When you turn off the visibility of a layer, it is still there, even though you can't see it.

Shamans drew or carved on rocks to draw out the spirit of the divine. It wasn't so much carving a pretty picture into a rock to admire for the art—like pinning a poster to your bedroom wall—but rather like creating a window into the spirit world for the divine to appear.

Another famous goddess image from that era is the goddess of Laussel, who was carved out of limestone on the wall at the entrance of a cave at Lascaux, France. Many beautiful paintings still adorn the walls of this cave, where people lived over 20,000 years ago. The goddess of Laussel is seventeen inches high and is painted red—the color of life-sustaining blood. She holds a bison's horn in her right hand shaped like a crescent moon, with thirteen notches carved along the curve. These notches represent the months of the year and women's menstrual cycles. They may have been a calendar for those ancient people.

Time, in those days, was thought of as cyclical rather than linear. Each year was like a spiral, passing through the four seasons in a circular fashion, bringing you back to the time of year you began your journey—only older and wiser. Life was a constant flow of waxing and waning, growth and decay, full and empty, seen and unseen; life, death, and rebirth. The seasons followed this pattern, as did the moon and women's cycles. All of life was seen to follow this pattern, and death was simply a birth into a different state of being.

··

Goddess Workout

Can you imagine living in a society where a goddess was the primary deity worshipped? Imagine people today still placed goddess statues outside their homes and carried little goddess amulets to protect them and remind them of their ability to give birth to their ideas, new life, and their creativity. These amulets would serve to show you that the Goddess was always there to sustain and nourish you. What would that be like? Would it change how you felt about being a girl in our society, do you think?

If large, voluptuous images of women were commonplace, would it make a difference in how you feel about your body?

Make your own goddess figurine out of modeling clay and paint it. If you like, make it in a shape that resembles your own body to remind you that you are a manifestation of the divine.

The Goddess in Neolithic Times

After the Paleolithic era came the Mesolithic era, from 8000 to 4000 B.C.E. Although we know these people were primarily food gatherers, like their predecessors, not much else is known about them, as they left very few traces of themselves behind. Next came the Neolithic era, from 4000 B.C.E. to 2000 B.C.E. People from this era left behind several thousand stone monuments, including Stonehenge, which were used as sacred ceremonial sites.

In the Neolithic era, people began to build more permanent bases instead of roaming the land as nomads. They learned how to farm and grow crops so they would not have to go searching for food so much. Now they depended greatly on the elements to nourish their food supply. These people worshipped the Goddess as the source of all water, from the rain that fell from the sky to the lakes and springs and rivers that welled up from within the Earth's body.

During this time people also worshipped the Goddess in the form of various animals. Birds were considered sacred to the Goddess because of their ability to travel effortlessly between the sacred realms of earth, sky, and water. The bird was an important figure in many ancient myths. Different cultures had creation myths that foretold of a great bird laying a cosmic egg from which the universe was born. The bird was also important because of its ability to signal weather patterns. Even today we know when the weather is getting colder or warmer when birds fly south and return.

The snake was another sacred goddess animal. She symbolized rebirth. The snake goddess was a powerful symbol of renewal. She could shed her skin and come forth from the womb of the Earth totally new. Many snake and bird goddess images appeared on vases at this time.

....

Goddess Workout

Close your eyes and go back in time, in your imagination, to when tribal people first walked the earth. Imagine you are one of those people. The Earth is your sacred mother. Feel your connectedness to her as part of your daily life. Every day you hunt for food from her body, drink water from her never-ending springs, and eat food from crops that spring forth from her body. Each night you sleep in a cave, enclosed in her womb. The sacred world is always at hand. You see the ancient wise ones in the trees, the rocks, the rivers, the stars. Everywhere you walk, you are aware that you are surrounded by allies from the invisible spirit world. Each day you commune with these wise ones, learning their secrets, sharing your thoughts.

You feel yourself being divinely guided through every step of your day. You know intuitively that you too are a spirit being, only on this earth for a short period of time, and that when you die you will be reborn back into the spirit realms. Each day you awaken with the expectancy that the goddess will provide for you exactly what you need for that day. Each dawn celebrates the birth of a new day—another opportunity to embrace the magic, the mystery, and the beauty of life. You give thanks each night for all that you have experienced.

Where Else Was She Worshipped?

Wherever people have lived on Earth, the Goddess has appeared—from Sumeria to Hawaii, Africa to America, and China to New Zealand. Writing about all the places where the Goddess was worshipped could fill a whole book. Such books already exist, like *The Myth of the Goddess* by Anne Baring and Jules Cashford (London: Viking, 1991), a 780-page volume on goddess worship throughout history.

Here I just provide a teaspoon of goddess history to give you an inkling of how goddesses have been important to many cultures.

In ancient Egypt, there were forty-two districts that each had their own gods and goddesses. Even little towns had a temple dedicated to their goddess or god. Later, when Egypt united, each region still revered their particular deity while other deities were worshipped throughout the land.

Early Egyptians thought the goddesses had bodies of birds or animals. There was the goddess Bastet, who took the form of a cat. She was worshipped as the goddess who brought sunlight to Earth. Thus cats were sacred in Egypt, and anyone who killed one would be sentenced to death.

Teweret was the goddess of childbirth, and she appeared as a pregnant hippopotamus! Egyptians believed the blood from her womb gave eternal life. As Egyptian society evolved, so, too, did the shapes the gods and goddesses took. Later Egyptians believed the goddesses had human bodies with animal heads. Some gods and goddesses were thought to appear entirely in human form. The most famous Egyptian goddess was Isis, goddess of love and destiny, whose worship continued under Roman rule. All the attributes of the many different Egyptian goddesses were present in her.

The Celtic people lived in central Europe and spread across the continent to France, Spain, Portugal, Turkey, England, Scotland, Wales, and Ireland. The Celts were linked because they shared similar languages but, unlike the Egyptians, they were never one nation with one leader. Nor did they worship all the same gods. Most of the different Celtic tribes had deities who were local to each area, just like the early Egyptians.

The cauldron was central to Celtic life and beliefs. The cauldron would hang from wooden rafters in the center of the house with a fire underneath, and it was the most important feature in the home. Celts used the cauldron to cook meals in and to boil water to wash with. The fire gave off light, which was important because there were no windows in Celtic houses, and heat to keep everyone warm.

In Celtic mythology, the cauldron represented abundance, fertility, and rebirth. It could also represent a woman's womb, which was another cauldron or container of fertility and birth. Again and again in history, the Goddess and her life-giving properties parallel with women's cycles.

There were many powerful goddesses in Celtic mythology and legend. The Morrigan was goddess of fertility and death. When she appeared during the summer months in her form as a raven, people knew death was near. When she appeared during the winter, she would bring signs of new life.

Queen Boadicea was a real woman who was the ruler of the Iceni tribe. When Romans raped her daughters, she gathered together people from lots of other tribes and led a revolt against the Romans. A powerful warrior, Queen Boadicea relied on her goddess power by invoking the goddess Andraste before each battle.

Brighid was the Celtic goddess of healing, poetry, and crafts. A flame for her still burns today in Kildare, Ireland. People all over the world keep a vigil over her sacred flame.

....

Goddess Workout

Check out the website dedicated to the flame of Brighid at:
http://ordbrighideach.org

In ancient Greece, temples were built as homes for the Greek goddesses and gods. The city of Athens was named for the goddess Athena, the goddess of wisdom. In her temple there was a magnificent statue of her, carved from ivory and gold. Today, the remains of her temple still stand above Athens.

The Greeks believed they could contact the goddesses and gods through prayer and sacrifice or by visiting an oracle where a priestess would advise them of the deity's will. Priestesses devoted to the Goddess served at her temples. People would visit the priestesses to receive the Goddess's blessings and petition requests. They would bring offerings to the Goddess in the form of food and coins.

Sacrifice was an important element of Roman tradition. Each temple in Rome was also dedicated to a particular god or goddess. Sacrifices were made to persuade a deity to grant a request.

Each family had their own home shrine where they gave daily offerings of incense, cakes, and wine to the household gods. The Penates were household deities who were the protectors of the storeroom. They were responsible for the family's wealth. The Lares brought the family prosperity and happiness. If you have seen the movie *Gladiator,* you may remember the small figurines that the gladiator carried with him and brought out when he prayed for his family. These were Lares.

In Roman households, the father was called the genius and the whole family, as well as the slaves, worshipped him. Everybody under Roman rule worshipped the emperor as the state genius. The Romans believed failure to worship their gods would lead to a disaster at home or for the entire empire.

In Rome, there were forty-five public holidays each year to celebrate various gods and goddesses. One such goddess was Vesta, the goddess of home and hearth. Her round temple in the Forum was one of the most important buildings in Rome. A sacred fire was kept burning there at all times, and priestesses called vestals tended the flame. Girls from noble families could become priestesses of Vesta and serve at her temple. To be her priestess was a great honor. But if a priestess disgraced the Goddess, she would be buried alive as punishment.

Goddess Workout

Make a shrine for a goddess in your bedroom. Place a picture or a statue of a goddess on your dresser. Tarot cards or angel figurines work well. Decorate your shrine with candles, flowers, perfume, glitter, shells, or anything you like.

Why Did the Goddess Seemingly Disappear?

By now you can see the Goddess was worshipped for many different reasons in many different cultures. She could bestow fertility, grant personal favors, and provide food and shelter in the form of plentiful crops, warm caves, or wood to build with. She could also grant requests in the nature of love, healing, and prosperity.

So if the Goddess was such an important figure to many races so long ago, why isn't she now? Well, the Goddess is still central to many religions around the world, but several events happened that changed the way people worshipped in the Western world.

Two important events that helped shape modern religious history were:

1. Rome conquered many countries, including the British Isles.

2. Christianity became the official religion of Rome.

There were many other events that contributed to the demise of goddess worship. During the Middle Ages there were witch hunts directed against women, and in the eighteenth century there were missions to the New World. During this time, as the British Empire grew, missionaries from England traveled to many countries, converting them to Christianity.

In the sixth century B.C., Rome was a magnificent city. The Romans gradually became powerful in other lands. They conquered tribes throughout Europe until by A.D. 117 the Roman Empire had reached its peak, spreading all the way from Britain to Egypt, and from Spain all the way across to the Middle East.

As the Roman Empire grew, many of the gods and goddesses from foreign lands that Rome claimed were still worshipped in their country of origin. Some, like Isis, became part of Roman beliefs. Mithras, the Persian god of light and war, was another foreign deity who was absorbed into Roman culture. He was especially popular with Roman soldiers. In London, there are remains of a temple built for Mithras.

In A.D. 324, the Emperor Constantine made Christianity the official Roman religion. Christianity was different from other religions at that time because it was based on the life and teachings of an actual person—Jesus of Nazareth. In Christianity there was only one male god—no goddesses. One of the basic premises of Christianity was "thou shalt have no other gods before me" (from the Ten Commandments in the Bible). Whereas before the religion of the Roman Empire was polytheistic, meaning there was a belief in many gods and goddesses, with the onset of Christianity it became monotheistic. Christians believed in only one god: God the father.

In Britain, when Christianity first arose, things did not change much. People thought the story of Mary being impregnated by God and giving birth to Christ was another variation of the goddess and her child. There were already many Pagan festivals of the Earth Goddess being impregnated by the Sun God and giving birth.

Beltane, May 1, was one festival when the fertility of the Earth Goddess was enacted. A maypole (representing the Sun God) was lowered into a hole in the earth (representing the Goddess). Once impregnated by the Sun God, the Earth Mother would hold his seed within her body and burst forth with new crops later in the year. The celebration at spring ensured the Earth's fertility and the Goddess's blessing on her people.

After the Romans left Britain, paganism returned. In Ireland, missionaries such as Patrick brought Christianity to the people. Their Christianity, which was later called Celtic Christianity, was different than the kind of Christianity the Romans had established. In the seventh century, Gregory the Great sent Augustine to the British Isles to convert people to the Roman style of Christianity.

During this time, Britain was about half Pagan and half Christian. But by the fourteenth century, Britain was now clearly Christian, and mistrust of women had become a major theme of Christianity. In 1484, Pope Innocent VIII launched an inquisition against the old Earth religions, the Goddess, and her followers, especially women (who were the female expressions of the Goddess).

In 1486, two Dominican monks wrote and published the *Maleus Malificarum (The Witches' Hammer)*, which stated women and their sex drive was pure evil: "All witchcraft stems from carnal lust which in women is insatiable."

The book gave ways to recognize, torture, and kill a woman who was considered a witch. Any woman could be labeled a witch by a jealous neighbor, a bitter ex-lover, or even a witch hunter trying to make more money. Women healers were especially vulnerable, as the *Maleus Malificarum* said women with strange and magical powers were in consort with the devil.

A high price was paid for the head of a witch. If the woman was unable to prove her innocence, she was tortured until she signed a confession. Those who confessed were strangled. If the woman protested and said she was innocent, she was burned alive.

The inquisition lasted until the middle of the eighteenth century. Thousands of innocent women were tortured and killed (read *Witchcraze: A New History of the European Witch Hunts* by Anne Llewellyn Barstow [HarperCollins, 1994] for more information). Children were not spared either as the people who were performing these murders said children inherited evil from their mothers.

During the eighteenth century, as the British Empire gained rule over the countries it had invaded, Christianity spread, too, and native religions were forbidden. In Australia, Aborigines worshipped such goddesses as Kunapipi, the mother goddess who formed the land from her body and made children, animals, and plants. In New Zealand, Maoris worshipped goddesses like Mahuika, the fire goddess, and Marama, the moon goddess. Today many native peoples practice Christianity. When I was a child, my Maori grandmother pretended she could not speak Maori because she had been punished at school when she did. Nowadays people are becoming more aware of the need to preserve ancient traditions.

The Goddess Today

Some religions still worship goddesses. Some never stopped! Some ancient religions are becoming popular again, and some new religions are springing up with an emphasis on the goddess.

Hinduism was the name given to describe a number of religions in India. Its roots go back thousands of years. Many goddesses are worshipped in Hinduism.

Sarasvati is the goddess of wisdom, learning, music, and the arts. She invented Sanskrit, the Hindu language. She is so beautiful that her husband, Brahma, grew three faces so he could see her from every side. Today students in India pray to her for help with their exams.

Buddhism celebrates goddesses such as Kuan Yin and Tara. Kuan Yin is the goddess of compassion and mercy. She is the patron goddess of all children. She can appear in many forms, some male and some female.

Buddhism traveled to Japan from China and is practiced alongside the older Japanese religion, Shintoism. The sun goddess Amaterasu is the most important of all the Shinto deities. Ten million people visit her shrine at Ise each year. Her symbol, the rising sun, appears on the Japanese national flag.

Religions from Africa, such as Santería, continue to worship goddesses. There is Oshun, the goddess of love and beauty, and Yemaya, the river goddess who had lots of children, all with different fathers, including the thunder god Shango.

Many old Earth religions have enjoyed a resurgence in the past few years. Pagans, Wiccans, and Druids all worship a goddess.

Sophia, the goddess of wisdom in the Kabbalah, is central to the Jewish wisdom, as is Queen Esther, whose festival is celebrated at Purim in February. Even Christianity has goddesses, although most Christians do not consider them deities. Mary, the beloved mother of Christ, is greatly adored by people all over the world, which certainly qualifies her as a goddess according to the dictionary definition.

Mary of Bethany has long been one of my favorite women in the Bible and could be considered a goddess of devotion. In some Christian groups there are ministers who pray to a mother-father god rather than just a father god.

You can tune into the Goddess no matter what your religion. All religions that I know of have at least one important female. Also, the Goddess can help you, regardless of what your religion is. She has no religious boundaries. You don't have to change your religion to access your own goddess power. Do what you feel comfortable with.

A Word on the Nature of the Goddess

We can learn a lot about the nature of the Goddess by studying nature. Ancient peoples thought of the Goddess as the Earth herself, as she who gave birth to the entire universe. How does the universe operate? What do you notice happening in nature? Here's what I see.

The Goddess:

- Likes stuff. Lots of stuff. You can tell that because she makes infinite varieties of things, like snowflakes or blades of grass and even stars. She doesn't just make one or two things, she makes zillions.

- Is prosperous. There is so much abundance in nature—lakes filled with fish, fields brimming with flowers, the sky bursting with stars.

- Has a keen eye for beauty. Everywhere you look in nature, you see beautiful colors, like a master artist putting his or her finishing touches perfectly across the canvas of the universe.

- Is inventive. Well, come on now, you must be pretty inventive to create the Earth and everything on it—not to mention the rest of the universe and goddess knows what else there is outside of the universe in other dimensions.

- Is divinely intelligent. Everything she creates works in perfect symmetry. Even as the universe expands at an incredible rate, it does so with perfect wisdom so that it can self-regulate without hurting itself.

- Loves to be creative.

- Loves to manifest her creativity. It's one thing to have wonderfully creative ideas and another to bring them into fruition. You can tell by looking around on this very physical planet and seeing products of her creativity.

- Is passionate. Think of the brewing of a storm, the explosion of thunder, the torrent of rain, the roar of wind.

- Has a big cleanup every now and then. Yes, even the Goddess spring-cleans. We see this in what we call devastating acts of nature. Even the Goddess knows you make way for the new by clearing out the old.

- Knows there is a time for everything—a time to be still and wait, to let things gestate, a time to be active, a down time, and an active time.

- Is kind and loving. How do I know this? Well, I just do, so you'll have to take my word for it. And after you have hung out with the Goddess for a while, you'll discover that for yourself, too.

Goddess Workout

Add some of your own observations about the nature of the Goddess.

How Can the Goddess Help You Today?

The Goddess can help you in any way possible, from the most mundane to the most magical! There is no task too small or too big for her.

Here are some of the things the Goddess can help you with:

- If you are struggling with poor self-esteem

- If you want to lose weight

- If you want more love in your life

- If you want a boyfriend

- If you are having a hard time at school

- If you are having problems with friends

- If you're lonely

- If your parents don't seem to understand you

- If you want to get into a certain college

- If you don't know what you want to do with your life

There is no limit to what the Goddess can or cannot do! All you need to do is ask, believe, and receive. It's that simple. Throughout this book you will learn specific ways to do just that. Which brings us to the next chapter. . . .

Magic
101

Magic is when the seemingly impossible happens. There is nothing airy-fairy about magic. Anyone can practice it by following certain magical principles.

The main premise of magic is that there is a force greater than yourself at work in the universe. This force is always available to you. By utilizing various techniques such as prayers, incantations, visualizations, meditations, and ceremonies, you can learn how to channel the creative energy of the universe to produce a desired result.

In ancient times, people practiced magic by calling on the powers of the invisible realms, the Goddess, their ancestors, and animal allies. They used the power of nature, the power of the seasons, the sun, moon, and stars for help. They were very in tune with the natural world and used their knowledge of how the world of nature worked to their advantage. They knew everything followed a certain rhythm of gestating, growing, blossoming, waning, and repose. There was a time and a season for all dreams and desires.

Today many people still practice magic on a regular basis. There are many magical paths in the Western world. There is the Hermetic path, which includes ceremonial magic, the Golden Dawn, the Rosicrucians, the Masons, and the Kabala.

There is the Native path, which includes all Earth-based religions such as Paganism, Wicca, Druidry, Celtic magic, and Celtic Christianity. Many modern religions, such as Christianity and Judaism, have magical teachings within their traditions. You don't need to belong to a certain religion to practice magic. Magic is universal and can be practiced within the framework of any spiritual path.

Magic is fun. Magic believes the impossible can happen. Magic is learning to expect the unexpected. It is easier to live a magical life than a mundane one, where you expect to have to go it all alone. You can use magic for anything and everything, from getting a pretty pink spring dress to finding the love of your life to discovering your true purpose.

Why Do People Practice Magic?

Living a magical, enchanted life is fun! When you begin practicing magic, you open up to the idea that there are unseen forces at work in your life helping you make your dreams come true. Coincidences, miracles, and synchronicities become a regular occurrence.

Magic is embracing life with an open heart and an open mind. You put your rational, realistic mind on hold and tune into your optimistic, hopeful voice: "Well, statistics say this may never work, but I'll give it a go anyway."

What Can Magic Do for You?

When you live a magical life:

- You expect help from unseen sources.

- You trust in the immense power of the universe.

- You believe your dreams can come true, even if you can't see a way to make them come true.

- You start taking small steps toward making your dreams a reality.

- You expect help from unexpected sources to bring your dreams to fulfillment.

- You know there are allies, angels, and helpers, both in the seen world and the unseen world, who will come into your life and help you.

- You trust the right people to show up at the right time.

- You know the universe's timing is perfect, and when one door closes another will open; therefore, you don't worry about the details, you work with the universe's agenda, trusting that everything happens in divine timing.

- You know that faith without action is meaningless, so you do whatever you can at your end and trust the Goddess to take care of the rest.

- You ask for help with anything and everything, from the minor to the major, knowing that the Goddess loves to help you with all aspects of your life.

Magic Can Be Fun

- You can do spells to get kisses from cute boys.

- You can pray for a pretty dress in your favorite color.

Magic Can Be Frivolous

- You can pray for silly things you secretly desire—like a bunch of flowers or a box of chocolates.

Creating Magic

Magic is a skill that can be learned, like any other skill. To become proficient simply requires regular practice.

To participate in the creation of magic requires the following beliefs:

1. That you are a spiritual being.

2. That there is a force greater than yourself at work in the universe.

3. That you can manifest your dreams with the help of this force.

You Are a Spiritual Being

It doesn't matter whether you practice any form of spirituality or not. You are and always have been a spiritual being—a human with a spiritual body. Or another way of looking at it is you are a spirit with a human body. Anyway, you are made from the same spiritual substance as the Goddess. The reverend at the church I attend says we are all projections of God. I like that analogy. So think of yourself as a projection of the Goddess!

Your spirit is your true inner essence, your inner goddess, which you will learn more about in the next chapter. This essence can never be destroyed and it is unique to you, just like your fingerprints. Your spirit is the part of you that existed before you were born and it is the part of you that will exist once you are physically gone. Your spirit contains the spark of divinity. Through your spirit, you can communicate with the divine. Some people can see the spirit emanating from the physical body. This light is commonly known as your aura.

There Is a Force Greater Than Yourself at Work in the Universe

Spiritual truths are spiritual truths and they exist whether you believe in them or not!

Unless you are an atheist, this concept will not be difficult to accept. Look around outside; what do you see? The sky, the earth, trees, flowers, plants, birds—where did they all come from? Why are we here? Those are the questions scientists and philosophers have been grappling with for years. To work magic, it is necessary to believe that some kind of power greater than a human one exists. Whatever you call this power is unimportant. You may call it Goddess, God, Great Spirit, Buddha, Krishna, Divine Intelligence, Universal Power, or even Frank! Whatever. Which leads us to the next step . . .

You Can Manifest Your Dreams with the Help of This Force

You may think that living in accordance with a greater power is simplistic. It is. That's the beauty of it. When we believe the universe will help us manifest our dreams, life becomes much easier.

When you try to go it alone, you can often feel frustrated, anxious, or as if you must manipulate events in order to produce a desired outcome. When you work in tune with the power of the universe, you can set your intentions, take right actions, and trust that the results will appear.

In ancient cultures, the Druid, priestess, or shaman of a tribe was greatly respected and held a position of utmost authority. This position was higher than the king or chief. The priestess worked with the forces of nature to produce good crops, increase fertility, foretell the future, and communicate with the spirit world. There was no distinction between the seen physical world and the unseen spiritual world. Practicing spirituality and magic was a part of daily life.

The Principles of Magic and How to Practice Them

Principle Number One: All Magic Begins in the Mind

Your imagination is the greatest magical tool you possess. Your imagination is your very own magic wand, for whatever you think about most often will eventually come to pass.

Everything began as a thought somewhere. Look around you, what do you see? Every single thing that you see began as a thought in someone's mind.

Since we are made in the same spiritual likeness as divinity or God/Goddess, then we can assume that all manifestations in the physical universe began as a thought in the divine mind.

In order for something to manifest in the physical world, you have to think it up in the mental world first. This is how you make an imprint in the spiritual universe that eventually will be developed as something physical on earth.

Use your imagination wisely. Focus on what you *want* to have in your life, not what you don't want. Remember that whatever you pay attention to grows. So put your attention on things that you do actually want to grow.

Know that thoughts become things.

What magic are you creating in your mind?

MAGICAL DAYDREAMING

Maybe you have been told daydreaming is a waste of time and something you shouldn't do. Well, let me tell you right now that daydreaming is one of the greatest gifts you can give yourself.

Why? Because when you daydream, you are setting your dreams up in the spiritual world. Pretty soon they will show up in your physical reality. This is the law of cause and effect. So daydream about how great you would like to be.

Metaphysical teacher Louise Hay says that what you are thinking about today will show up in your life in six months' time. I usually find what I think about shows up a lot sooner than that—sometimes almost instantly.

The difference between magical daydreaming and regular daydreaming is with magical daydreaming you call on the Goddess for help. See her in your daydreams helping you and guiding you.

Magical daydreaming is like using your magic wand. Let me give you an example of how magical daydreaming has worked for me.

When I was twenty-two, I wanted to be an esthetician. However, there were no esthetician schools or licenses in New Mexico, where I lived. If you wanted to work as a skin-care specialist or makeup artist, you had to go to cosmetology school for nine months. One month focused on skin care and makeup, the rest on hair. Well, I wanted to go to the Aveda School in Minneapolis and take their esthetician program, which was six months of skin care, makeup, and aromatherapy, all taught from a holistic viewpoint. My rational mind said, "You're crazy! Why spend all that time and money to go when you won't even be able to work when you get back?" But I felt guided to go anyway. My inner voice said, "Go. Get the training. Deal with the licensing stuff when you get back." I felt the Goddess prompting me.

So off I went and I had a great time and learned lots of wonderful stuff. While I was gone, the local government introduced a licensing procedure for estheticians in New Mexico. When I returned, I was able to practice freely—no sweat. "Thank you, Goddess!"

I use magical daydreaming every day for big things and little things. Wonderful happenings are a regular occurrence in my life—and they can be for you, too!

What are you thinking about today?

Principle Number Two: What You Put Out Is What You'll Get Back

This is the law of cause and effect—what goes around comes around, whatever you put out comes back to you threefold—these are just various ways of stating the law of cause and effect. For every action there is a reaction.

27

The law of cause and effect is like the great big cosmic kitchen where you place your order and pretty soon your meal arrives. The law of cause and effect is the process that causes thoughts to manifest into things. The universe is impartial to our requests. It works perfectly every time. That means, like a great big mirror reflecting back our desires to us, it will give us whatever we believe to be true.

Thoughts have energy. Worry thoughts and fear-filled thoughts are like bubbles of smog and dust, whereas happy, successful, and love-filled thoughts are like bubbles filled with sparkles. Thoughts become things through the principle of cause and effect. When you think certain thoughts repeatedly, you are planting a seed in the spiritual world that will bloom in the physical world.

Look at your life right now. Are there any conditions or situations (effects) that you would like to change? If so, great! The way to change them is to start thinking of what you would like to experience instead. Before you can experience something in the physical world, you must first set it up in the spiritual world. Create a mental picture. If you keep holding that picture in your mind, you will find the divine mind will bring it to life.

Principle Number Three: Like Attracts Like

This is the law of correspondence. What are you attracting into your life? How would you like that to change?

Have you ever wondered why kids who seem unmotivated at school hang out with other kids who are not very motivated? Or why all the brainy kids seem to hang out together? This is because of principle number three—like attracts like. We automatically gravitate toward people, places, and things that vibrate at the same "vibe" as us.

I used to hang out with people who did a lot of drugs because at one time I thought that was cool. When I realized I wanted something more from my life, I naturally started to gravitate toward people who were also achieving more.

People who think selfish thoughts and act in selfish ways will attract more of the same to them. People who act with good intentions and put a lot of love out into the universe will find themselves surrounded by a lot of people who love them. If you want more love or faith or prosperity, or any other quality in your life, start acting that way first. Act loving and you will receive love; step out in faith and you will experience faith; act prosperous and you will become prosperous.

If you give out bad things, you will get bad experiences back

When you put out good things, you will get good experiences back

Principle Number Four: We Live in a Spiritual World

Our universe is a spiritual universe, and we are spiritual beings. There is a spiritual power that fuels our world and you can use this power to affect great changes in your life. Sometimes people dismiss spiritual power because they can't see it. This is crazy. Just because you can't see something does not mean it doesn't exist. Like oxygen, for example, or electricity—can you see those? Do you doubt their existence? If not, then it won't be too hard for you to make the leap in thinking that there is a spiritual power available for you to use, too. You will learn more about this great spiritual power in the chapter on "conjuring your destiny."

How You Can Tune Into the Forces of Nature for Help

Our lives are ruled by the forces of nature. Even though most of us do not live in such close contact with nature as our ancestors from the Stone Age did, we are still affected by it. We are affected by the magnetic pull of the moon, by the rhythm of the seasons, by the time of day, and by so many things that we take for

28

granted. There are many natural forces surrounding us that affect us. Have you ever noticed that a different season or a certain time of day affects you in a specific kind of way?

I always feel happy in spring. I love seeing the new life all around me, flowers springing up in my garden, tiny green leaves on the trees, little lambs and calves. Spring reminds me that darkness and chill always give way to warmth and hope. In ancient times, people worked with the natural world, the seasons, the moon, and the time of day. They called on the powers of the natural world for help, too. The power of the sun, the power of the moon, the power of the ocean, the power of the mountains—since everything is made from the same spiritual substance, all these things contain great spiritual power.

Your Magical Toolbox

Here are some tools that you may find useful to help you in your practice of magic. If you use them regularly, I promise you that your life will become more magical.

Affirmations

Affirmations are statements you make about yourself, your life, and your beliefs about the world. Affirmations can be positive or negative, depending on what kind of statement you make. We are constantly making affirmations throughout the day. Listen to conversations of people around you and take note of what they say. Words are very revealing as to people's belief systems and what they think is possible or not.

Affirmations are very powerful because they send a message to the universe as to what you want to order for your life. Every time you say something (out loud or in your mind), you are sending the universe your order. Imagine you are at a drive-through fast-food place speaking into the order box. This is what happens when you say anything. The universe gets the order, then begins to make the delivery.

What kind of affirmations are you saying throughout the day? Carry a card around with you for one week that says, "What am I saying to myself right now?"

Look at it regularly throughout each day and notice what your current thoughts or conversations are. Is what you are saying either to yourself or to another person something that you really want to be true for you? If not, then start reframing your language and thoughts into things that you *do* want to be true.

Meditation

Meditation is a tool you can use to get in touch with the spiritual nature of the universe and everything in it, including yourself. In meditation, you realize your divinity, you access your goddess power, and you commune with the Goddess and your inner holy spirit. There are many different forms of meditation. Experiment with different kinds until you find one that works for you.

I like guided meditation. And I like to use meditation tapes. They are very helpful for changing your consciousness and increasing your self-confidence, if you use them often. If you use a meditation tape every morning and every evening for a month, you will see definite results in the quality of your life. My personal favorites are *Chakra Clearing* by Doreen Virtue, *Morning and Evening Meditations* by Marianne Williamson, and *Morning and Evening Prayers and Meditations* by Joan Borysenko.

Prayers

Prayers are conversations with divinity. You can pray to any deity, saint, ascended being (like Jesus or a bodhisattva, for example), and, of course, to any goddess or your holy spirit. Two ingredients are important when praying. One is a specific intent—you know what you are praying for—and the other is the belief that the Goddess can and will make it happen. Here is a formula for effective prayers.

This formula is for any type of prayer you use. You also can use this format for regular prayers, spells, or ceremonies. The only difference when you do a spell or ceremony is that you will be using sacred objects like candles, food, or crystals. This is how magical prayer works:

1. Ask for what you want

2. Visualize the outcome

3. Expect results

4. Let it go

5. Give thanks

ASK FOR WHAT YOU WANT

Write down what you want on a piece of paper, or have a conversation in your mind with the Goddess about what you want. Tell her exactly what it is that you want. Don't worry about how impossible it may seem. Remember, magic is when the seemingly impossible happens.

VISUALIZE THE OUTCOME

See yourself as having exactly what it is that you asked for. See the Goddess helping you to achieve it. See the Goddess sending angels and people and messages to guide you. See her opening doors where you thought there were no doors. Imagine how you will feel when you have the answer to your prayer. Spend time daydreaming about it—how good you will feel, how happy you will be. Imagine it is already happening right now. You see, your brain cannot differentiate between experiences that are happening and things that you vividly imagine. The more that you vividly imagine something, the more you bring it into being.

··

Goddess Workout

Make a symbol to represent the outcome. For example, if you want to be a rock star or start a band, make a CD cover. If you want a car, get a little Matchbox car to represent what you want. If you want a boyfriend, make a collage and cut pictures from magazines that show the qualities he has.

EXPECT RESULTS

Trust that the Goddess is already answering your prayers. You have put your order into the divine kitchen, and now it is being cooked up for you and will soon be delivered. Keep expecting it to show up. Say affirmations, like "My boyfriend is on his way to me now" or "I now have this great new car." Know that on the spiritual plane you do already possess those things, and you are just waiting for them to manifest on the physical plane.

Trust that the right doors will open at the right time and that the right answers will be given. The right people will cross your path. Take any necessary actions that you can—the Goddess will guide you with this. Keep your eyes open for the hand of the Goddess and the angels helping you.

LET IT GO

This means you know that the Goddess is working on it, so you don't have to spend any time fretting or worrying about it. I have a poster in my kitchen that reminds me of this. It says:

Good morning, this is God

I will be handling all your problems today

I do not need your help

So don't worry about anything

Just have a great day

You might like to write that quote down on a piece of paper and include a line underneath "I will be handling all your problems" to say something about your prayer being taken care of, like "I am bringing you your new car" or "I have found the perfect boyfriend for you and he will be there shortly"—something like that!

GIVE THANKS

The Goddess and the angels love to help us. All of divinity loves to help us. It is our birthright to be happy and prosperous. Living in misery and lack serves no one. So when you get the answer to your prayers, give thanks. You can even give thanks *before* you see the results showing up in your life, just as a way to remind yourself they are on their way. Say something like, "I give thanks for the perfect boyfriend, who is coming into my life now!"

....

Goddess Workout

Answered prayers—an exciting experiment! Now we are going to put our formula into action. Choose one thing you would like to resolve or manifest at this time. Write it down in your goddess journal. Start a letter: *Dear Goddess* . . . and tell her exactly what you would like. Then follow the steps outlined above, writing them down, too, in your journal, if you want. Date the letter and put it away for two weeks. Then go back to your journal and write about the results that have shown up so far. Keep visualizing the outcome and doing your magical daydreaming until your prayer comes true.

Spells, Ceremonies, and Rituals

Spells, ceremonies, and rituals are prayers with props. The universe loves symbolic gestures. A spell can be as simple as lighting a candle and saying a prayer. Or you can do an elaborate ritual where you set up sacred space and prepare a beautiful meal to honor divinity. Using magical tools and taking the time to do a ceremony helps the mind to focus. You learn how to make the mundane sacred.

Everyone has rituals they perform on a daily basis: brushing your teeth after dinner, making your bed before school, or buying a magazine each week from a newsstand. Think of a ritual you perform regularly.

There are still occasions when we perform ceremonies in our society. Funerals, weddings, birthdays, retirements, and christenings are a few examples. During a ceremony you invite others to come together to mark the occasion. When you do a sacred ceremony you are setting a special intention to acknowledge the presence of divinity and to ask for a blessing or help with your undertaking.

How to Have a Magical Day

* Set your intentions for the day every morning.

* Pray to the Goddess to be with you and help you take guided action.

I first learned how to have a magical day from my dad, who was a master of magic (although he wouldn't use quite those words!). My dad always said, "You have to get up every morning and say to yourself out loud: Today is going to be the best day of my life! And then you set about making that happen."

That's what my dad did every day. He went from growing up in a house of poverty—where there was no bathroom, no toilet, hardly any money, and scarce food—and being forced to leave school when he was thirteen because there was no money in his family. And he went on to become a very successful businessman and one of the richest men in his town, owning his own company and employing many people.

You see, my dad knew the power of believing, of imagining, and of taking right action.

So get up each morning and set your intentions for the day. Intend to have a magical, joyous day and mentally see yourself doing just that. See the Goddess helping you.

Each morning I write my intentions for the day in my day planner. Today I wrote:

* I intend to think good things about me.

* I intend to think good things about Stephen.

* I intend to think GREAT things about our marriage.

* I intend to eat one plum, some watermelon, and half a banana (I haven't been remembering to eat fruit lately).

* I intend to drink one bottle of water.

* I intend to read about Aphrodite and Psyche and make notes.

- I intend to go to a bookstore.

- I intend to finish my romance writers speech.

- I intend to HAVE FUN!!!!

You have the power to make each day as happy and as magical as possible, and to call on the Goddess for help.

Goddess Workout

Write down your intentions for the rest of your day now.

Further Reading

The Mental Equivalent by Emmet Fox

The Kybalion: Hermetic Philosophy by Three Initiates

Make every day magical!

Awakening Your Inner Goddess

Who Is Your Inner Goddess?

Your inner goddess is your divine self. She is unique to you. You carry the divine wisdom of the Great Goddess within you. You are made from the same spiritual substance as the Great Goddess, but how you manifest your divinity is unique. Your inner goddess is the Great Goddess expressing herself as you! Everybody has an inner goddess or an inner god. This is your wise, divine self. How you express your divinity will be different from anyone else on the planet.

How Can You Contact Her?

The best way to contact your inner goddess is by getting quiet. Lock yourself in your bathroom, if you have to, but find a quiet place where you won't be disturbed. Every day, spend ten minutes dwelling on your goddess nature. I like to do this at night in bed before I go to sleep.

First Focus on the Goddess

Close your eyes. Gently push all thoughts of any problems or distractions gently out of your mind. Bring a picture of the Goddess into your imagination. See her in all her radiance before you.

Expand Your Focus to the Magnificent Power of the Goddess

Now think about how powerful the Goddess is. Think about how powerful divine wisdom is. Think about how she created the universe perfectly, and everything in the universe perfectly. Think about how she has an unlimited supply of creativity, love, intelligence, and beauty. Think about how there is no problem too big or too small for the Goddess. There is nothing she can't help you with. Nothing.

Realize That You Are Made from This Power

Remember that we are all made from the same spiritual substance, so start thinking about how the same divine intelligence that created the universe created you. Think about all the amazing things this divine intelligence does for you every day. Divine power is the intelligence that causes your heart to beat, your lungs to breathe, your hair to grow, and your body to function—all without you having to think about it or do anything. Divine intelligence causes babies to grow in their mother's wombs without the mother having to do anything.

Think about how your divine nature is made up of goddess nature. We all carry the wisdom of the ancient goddess within us. Since at one time the Goddess has been worshipped in every single continent in one form or another, it is very likely that one of your ancestors worshipped a goddess. One of your ancestors may well have been a priestess of the Goddess. At the very least, you come from a lineage where people felt attuned with the spiritual world. No matter what culture or belief system you come from, if you go back far enough, you will eventually trace your heritage back to people who lived in tune with the natural world.

Realize this wisdom still runs in your veins via your DNA.

Acknowledge Your Divinity

Knowing all the things divine power is capable of doing, we can deduce that divine power is intelligent, creative, and powerful. This power is within you. You are a perfect manifestation of the divine. Divine power, divine intelligence, divine wisdom, divine beauty, and divine love radiate through you. When you live from your spirit, you are directed by an inner knowing at all times.

Your inner goddess is not concerned with the things your personality worries about. She knows there is a divine plan for your life. Your inner goddess is filled with perfect love and perfect trust. Therefore, the more in tune you are with your inner goddess, the more you live from your spirit and the more magical your life becomes. You are filled with peace, love, joy, beauty, and wisdom. You have a quiet calm about you, knowing every step you take is guided and in perfect harmony with the spirit of the goddess. Fears and doubts slip away and an inner confidence takes their place. You begin to see yourself as you truly are: a divine expression of the Goddess.

There is an innate perfection in your inner goddess. She is utterly unique and utterly you. Your inner goddess is the Goddess expressing herself through you.

Now say: "I, (your name), know that the Goddess is expressing herself in me, (your name). I know that I am a perfect manifestation of the Goddess. Divine intelligence, divine power, divine love, divine beauty, and divine wisdom are available to me right now. The power of the Goddess flows through me."

Have a Conversation with Your Inner Goddess

Now is the time to bring up all your worries, fears, and doubts. Tell your inner goddess exactly what is going on with your life. She already knows anyway, because she is omniscient (all-knowing). This is also the place to bring up your dreams and desires. See your life unfolding exactly the way you would like it to. See yourself achieving your heart's desires. See yourself safe, loved, and protected, at home in the arms of the Goddess. Ask the Goddess what you need to do today. Just say: "What one thing do I need to do, Goddess?"

Spend the next few minutes listening to her answer. Write it in your goddess diary.

How Will Your Inner Goddess Contact You?

Your inner goddess talks to you through your mind. That is why it is so important to spend some time every day being quiet so you can hear her. When you pray, you are having a conversation with the Goddess. A conversation implies communication between two or more. Therefore, it stands to reason that the Goddess will talk back to you—otherwise you would just be talking at the Goddess.

How does she talk to you? Through your intuition, your dreams, your gut feelings, and your inner promptings. That is why it is crucial that you get quiet so you can pay attention to your inner voice.

The Goddess talks to you through your mind by giving you clarity, insight, and realizations. When you have an "aha" moment, this is the voice of the Goddess. She will also give you inspiration and divine ideas. You will begin to think of creative solutions to problems you have. Divine energy begins as mental energy. You basically have a telepathic conversation with the Goddess.

How do you know when it is the Goddess talking to you, and you are not just making it up? The more you practice, the more accustomed you will become at discerning your human voice from your inner goddess's voice. A good rule of thumb is that your inner goddess always comes from a place of love and a place of possibility. She is not ruled by fear or limitation, as we humans sometimes are. If a fear thought comes to you, then you know that is not your inner goddess talking. Fear thoughts often begin with "I can't . . . I'm scared . . . There's no way . . . It's impossible . . . There's not enough . . ."

Once you start getting inner promptings, begin following them and see where they lead. Start acting as if you are divinely guided at all times. During the day, remind yourself that your inner goddess is directing you right now. Sometimes you will get divine messages from situations or people around you. For example, one Thursday night I awoke at 3 A.M. feeling anxious and upset. I pulled out my copy of *The Artist's Way* and began reading it. As I read, I began talking to the Goddess; I said, "I wish Julia Cameron (the author) still taught classes and I could go to one. She's so wise." The next day my friend Maya came over for dinner.

"Julia Cameron is teaching a class here," she told me.

"I have to go," I blurted out, telling Maya about my wish from the night before.

Then I gathered all the necessary information to enroll, but my rational human mind was throwing a bucket of cold water over the whole thing. "It's too expensive; who's going to take care of your boys; you can just read her book, you don't need to go." However, my inner goddess kept prompting me to go. Fortunately I know enough about divine guidance to turn my rational voice down and act on my goddess promptings. That's where the magic is.

Here is a meditation to help you tune into your inner goddess.

Meditation to Meet Your Inner Goddess

Read through this meditation once or record it before beginning.

Set up sacred space if you wish. Light a candle, put some soothing music on the stereo, burn some incense.

Lie down, close your eyes, just relax.

Say a prayer: "Goddess, guide me as I take this journey to meet my inner goddess."

Now imagine you are at your favorite place in nature. This can be a place that exists that you have been to before, a place that you have seen on TV or in a travel magazine, or it can be a place that is in your imagination.

Use all your senses to see this place. Look around you—what do you see? Listen—what do you hear? Notice how the place feels and what you can smell. Spend a minute here just enjoying the peace and solitude. Allow your body to fully relax into the beauty of this place.

Now begin walking in your imagination. Continue walking until you come to a tree—a very large tree. As you get closer, you notice a doorway in the tree. The doorway has magical symbols on it. You open the door. It is quite heavy but still you manage to open it without too much effort.

Inside the tree it is very dark. There is a sliver of light that comes through from the top of the tree. As your eyes grow accustomed to the dark, you notice there is a full-length mirror in front of you. You feel yourself being pulled toward this mirror. Slowly you walk forward until you are almost touching the mirror. Then an indescribable force pulls you closer.

You feel your body being pulled upward, higher and higher, through a whirling, swirling vortex of energy. The energy is both gentle and forceful. You feel calm and expectant. Higher you go, up past the tree, through the sky and the stars, until you are moving so fast your vision becomes a blur.

Finally you land with a thump on the ground. You know without a doubt you are in the enchanted realm of the Goddess. You look around you. Everything here is so beautiful. You take a moment to absorb the beauty of your surroundings. Here you feel perfectly at home, safe and secure. There is a lightness of being to you here. You feel the perfect wisdom and love of the place emanating around you and through you.

After a while, you notice a woman sitting on the ground before you. She is the most beautiful woman you have ever seen. She has the kindest eyes imaginable, and there is a glow about her. You know without a doubt that you are in the presence of the Goddess, she who created the bounty and beauty of the universe. She smiles at you and holds out her hand. You take her hand. "My daughter," she says. "Tell me what is on your heart." You begin to talk to her, telling her whatever you wish.

She strokes your hair and your shoulders and then places her hand over your heart. "My child," she says, "my love, beauty, and wisdom flow through you, for we are made of the same substance. Thou cometh from me. You are my precious daughter and how precious you are. Divine love fills you, divine wisdom guides you, and divine beauty surrounds you. Feel now the power of your goddess self."

She holds her hands on you for several minutes and you feel yourself being charged with the power of the Goddess. Then she hands you a mirror. "Look, my child—this is your goddess self, this is your spirit self. You have the power to create whatever you wish for your life. My divinity flows through you. I am always with you. There is never a moment in your life when I am not there, whether you realize it or not. I am always with you and through me all things are possible. Trust me, my child. Give your struggles to me that I may uplift you, give your dreams to me that I may enable you, let your vision be clear so you may see yourself as you truly are: pure spirit, goddess made manifest." She holds the mirror in front of you with one hand. Her other hand is pressed firmly against your back. "Thou art Goddess," she instructs. "Never forget that."

42

As you gaze into the mirror, you see clearly your goddess self. The image becomes clearer and clearer until you can see without a doubt your spirit self, your goddess self. This is the self you want to bring more of into the world.

Spend a few minutes connecting with your inner goddess. Ask her questions; you can ask the Goddess sitting beside you questions, too. When you have said everything you need to, look into your goddess self's eyes and ask her what one thing you need to do at this time to bring more of her into your mundane being. When she gives you an answer, thank her. Now it is time for you to leave, but you do not feel sad because you know she is within you at all times and you can connect to her whenever you need to. You get ready to make the journey back to the physical world.

Slowly begin to come back to this room, this time, this place. Become aware of where your body is lying; gently move your legs, your arms, and your head. Slowly open your eyes and bring your consciousness into this room. When you are ready, make notes in your goddess diary about your experience.

Give Your Inner Goddess a Name

Names have power. Giving your inner goddess a name is important because it will empower you to start seeing yourself in a different way. Your inner goddess name is your magical name—a name to remind you that you are a magical, divine being. This is the self that you want to bring more of into the world.

Remember, your magical name is your personal name of power. You don't have to share it with anybody. In some magic circles, people's magic names are only to be used within the circle. In some traditions people come out with their names because they want others to see them differently. It is probably a good idea to keep your name to yourself at first, as you work on developing your goddess power. Other people's negative comments or jokes can undermine your confidence in the early stages.

Think about the qualities of your goddess self. Think carefully about the kind of name you would like to have. This will be your secret name to symbolize your magical personality. How do you choose a name? You can find a name in all sorts of places. You could choose to take on the name of a goddess, an ancestor, some-one you admire, or a quality you wish to express.

Names have great power. They conjure up images of different qualities. You probably already associate names with different personality traits, based on people you have already known or your own personal bias. Television actors, celebrities, or characters from books can also affect the way we think about certain names. For example, when you think of the name Britney, who springs to mind?

If you don't believe that names have power, read the following names and see what kind of picture springs into your mind.

Jessica

Willard

Brad

Molly

Summer

What about your given name? Do you like the name your parents gave you or not? Do you know why they named you that? Are you called by your full name or an abbreviation? Do you have nicknames? Are they complimentary or derogatory? Even nicknames said in a jokey way can stick with you if they sound mean. One of my friends in high school was called Stick because she was thin and tall. The boys were relentless in their teasing, although I'm sure they didn't intend to be mean. Every day would be a chance for a new joke. "I'm going to *branch* off here," they'd say as they walked away from her, or "*Leaf* your book on the table"—anyway, you get the picture.

If you have never liked your given name, you may choose to change it as you get older. I know several women who have done this to great effect. A new name can change how you see yourself.

Remember, your magical name may change over time to reflect changes within yourself. You might like to change it every year on your birthday to bring out a different aspect of yourself.

I have had many different magical names along the way. When I was four I used to call myself Daffodil because I loved daffodils. They were bright, sunshiney flowers and I suppose in a way I wanted to be a bright, sunshiney child, because I was quite shy. As I got older I did, in fact, become more outgoing. As a preteen I would secretly call myself Gloria and pretend I was a glamorous sixteen-year-old.

A recent magical name I gave myself is Grania. Grania is a sun goddess in the Celtic tradition. It is also the name of Grania Ni Mhaille, a Celtic warrior woman who lived at the same time as Queen Elizabeth I. Grania was a feisty, strong, determined woman who was confident of her own power—qualities I wanted to display. Plus, Anne is my given middle name, and Aine (the Celtic version of Anne) is a derivative of Grania.

Create a Goddess Persona

Your goddess persona is your goddess personality. What kind of traits would you like your goddess personality to have? As you read through this book and learn about all the different goddesses, you will become more aware of the very many different strengths each one has. You too have your own special, unique goddess traits. Your goddess personality can be as magical and enchanted as you wish it to be. What are some of the qualities that you have perhaps admired in other people and would like to cultivate yourself? I always used to admire people who were strong and could stand up for themselves. I used to shrink from confrontation and at the first sign of an upset begin apologizing, whether it was my fault or not. So I decided I wanted more "kick butt" attitude in my goddess persona.

Become aware in your imagination of what you want your goddess persona to appear like. The more you live from your goddess center, the more you realize you don't have to cower before anyone. You can hold your head up high, throw your shoulders back, and proudly announce to the world, "I am a daughter of the Goddess." In fact, whenever I get a panic attack of inferiority for any reason, that is exactly what I do.

....

Goddess Workout

Stand up tall. Walk to the nearest mirror and say, *"I, (your name), am a daughter of the Goddess. The blood of the Goddess flows through my veins. The power of the Goddess flows through my veins. I can do all things through the power of the Goddess."*

Write a list of goddess qualities you want to incorporate into your magical personality.

Each morning mentally see yourself as having those goddess qualities. Spend five minutes before you get out of bed picturing yourself as a goddess.

What kind of goddess would you like to be? A goddess of love, a goddess of battle, a goddess of healing?

What kind of goddess would you like to help you?

Once you have your goddess persona clear in your mind, you can invoke a goddess to help you carry it out. This way you are plugging in to the divine power that is available to us all.

Remember, there are many different goddesses from many different cultures, as we talked about earlier. Later in this book you will meet specific goddesses and learn more about them in further detail. You can ask for guidance from a particular goddess or from divine spirit, or even from God or a particular god from another culture. It is totally up to you and what you feel comfortable with.

If you could see yourself in any way possible, how would you most like to see yourself? Make this as elaborate and detailed as you can. Hold nothing back. Perhaps you have always thought of yourself as unattractive and have wished that you were prettier. Write down exactly how pretty you would like to be and start mentally seeing yourself that way. Call on a goddess of beauty, such as Aphrodite, to help you. If you are struggling with exams, call on a goddess of study, like Lakshmi. See yourself studying diligently and getting great grades.

Once you have this information, you can decide what kind of goddess you need to invoke to help you with your goddess persona. If you don't know of a particular goddess who could help your present situation, don't worry. You'll learn more about different goddesses and their areas of specialty in the second part of this book. In the meantime, just pray to "goddess of healing" or "goddess of beauty" or "goddess of all." You could even choose to pray to a modern goddess, like "goddess of rock-and-roll" or "goddess of the Web." Remember, there is no limiting the Goddess. She has shown up in many forms and faces throughout history, so there is no reason why she shouldn't keep doing so. You can see her however you choose.

47

When you are ready to invoke a goddess, just close your eyes, ask the Goddess to fill you with her divine energy, and visualize this taking place.

Goddess Workout

For one day, pretend you are the goddess of _____ (you choose). Live and act as the goddess of your choice. When you get into a situation that you are not sure how to deal with, ask yourself, "How would the goddess of _____ act?" Then act accordingly.

Make a Goddess Shrine

A goddess shrine is a special place set aside especially for communion with the Goddess. I have several friends who have entire rooms just for this purpose. As a mother of two small boys, I don't have that much space, so my goddess shrine is on my dressing table. If you have your own bedroom, you could turn it into your very own goddess temple. You could get ideas from pictures of goddess temples from ancient times or you could design your own modern-day temple. Hang goddess pictures on the walls, place candles around the room, keep sacred objects on your dressing table, and create a room worthy of a goddess residing there.

If, like me, you don't have much space, use a dressing table, mantelpiece, or a corner of a room. Put special, goddessy things in your shrine. If you are working with a particular goddess, include objects that are sacred to that goddess. When I make a shrine to honor Aphrodite, I use roses, pink candles, wine or sparkling grape juice, beautiful shells, pearls, perfume, and even lipstick (well, she is the goddess of beauty). Ask your goddess what she would like on her altar.

What about if you don't have much privacy and don't want anyone to see your shrine? Use a shoebox to store an altar cloth and special objects in. Then take them out when you are alone and use them when you pray. You can have your own traveling goddess shrine, just like the people from the Stone Age. Remember how they used to carry goddess figurines among their work tools?

A place in nature or a certain sanctuary may also be somewhere you communicate with the goddess. You may already have a special place that serves as a goddess shrine for you. In my hometown there is a water hole in a river known locally as the Big Black Hole. For years I would go there to renew my spirit. In New Mexico there is a Catholic shrine to Mary tucked away in the old town plaza that I like. The ancient Druids had no temples or shrines to worship in. They preferred to use groves of trees as their sacred places.

Make a Mandala of Your Goddess Self

A goddess mandala is a sacred picture of your goddess self. Use your mandala to meditate on, as a sacred vision of what you are in the process of becoming. Therefore, the images and symbols you use in your mandala need to reflect what you wish to become. What you need is a blank piece of cardboard, some magazines, colored pens, scissors, glue, stickers, and glitter. Draw a large circle almost to the edges of your cardboard. Inside the circle you are going to put all the different things your inner goddess likes. Include anything and everything—favorite fashion styles, colors, textures, makeup, and food. You can also use pictures of actual goddesses or tarot cards. But be careful if you use models or celebrities—the point is to emphasize your own divinity and uniqueness, not to become a carbon copy of someone else. Plus I don't want you to set unrealistic expectations for yourself of what you "should" look like.

Your mandala can be a great place to include pictures of what you would like to bring into your life. For example, if you have a secret dream to be a writer, then include something to symbolize that. You could draw a picture of a book, cut out a photo of some pens and paper, or create a writer costume for yourself. You may be surprised to find yourself putting in colors you have never worn before or styles that you usually shy away from. Allow yourself to experiment and be open to the emergence of a new you.

Cut out your mandala and hang it where you will see it regularly. You don't need to tell anyone what it is. Every time you look at it, remind yourself that this is what you are in the process of becoming. This is your true spiritual state.

49

Goddess Workout

Spend some time getting to know your inner goddess this week. Ask her questions. What kinds of food does she like to eat? How does she like to be treated? What kinds of hobbies does she like? What kinds of clothes does she like? What does she like to do for fun? Build up a picture of her in your imagination each night before you go to sleep. Make her as radiantly beautiful as you can, and ask her for guidance and suggestions.

A Sacred Ceremony to Honor Your Goddess Self

This is a fun ceremony that you can do over and over, whenever you want. You can do it when you need a self-esteem boost, before a date, on your birthday, or just for fun. I like to do it on a Friday night because Friday is sacred to Aphrodite, my patron goddess. Friday is ruled by Venus, the Roman goddess of love and beauty, and is a great time for any love magic or beauty magic. However, any night will work. You could also try doing a mini-version of it each morning, as you get ready for your day.

What you will need:

- ◆ Your goddess name

- ◆ A candle

- ◆ A goddessy costume

- ◆ Makeup, jewelry

- ◆ Your goddess mandala or a picture of the Goddess

- ◆ A mirror

- ◆ Good food

- ◆ Bubble bath

- ◆ Essential oil or perfume

- ◆ Body oil

- ◆ A quiet hour

- ◆ A bathroom

Step One: Getting Ready

Begin planning this ceremony a day in advance so you can gather up all that you need. For food you just need a couple of things. Bread and milk sweetened with honey are sacred to the Goddess. If you would rather have something else, go for it. A piece of cake or a couple of cookies are good, too. Make sure you get something you really like. You are the one who will be eating it and this is a celebration.

Get a candle in your favorite color.

For your goddessy costume, you don't need to go out and buy a whole new outfit. You can use whatever you have. A favorite outfit is perfect, as are dressing gowns, nightdresses, long flowing gowns, or jeans and a T-shirt. You have to decide what you want your inner goddess to look like. You may like to use temporary tattoos, glitter, and sparkly hair barrettes.

What if you don't feel very good about the way you look and don't think you will look good in anything? That's a common problem. Don't worry, we will cover beauty magic in the chapter on Aphrodite. For now, just ask the Goddess for help. She loves you just the way you are and can already see your divine beauty. Think of yourself as a goddess-in-training.

Some women have special goddess costumes that they only wear when performing goddess magic. You might like to have a special outfit, too. I don't have any clothes that I set aside especially for magic. My motto is "Make every day magical," so I like to pretend *all* my clothes are goddess clothes.

Gather up all your stuff and lock yourself in the bathroom. You will be in there for a while, so it's best to make sure no one else at home will be wanting to use it.

Now run the water and fill the bathtub. Add your bubble bath and a couple drops of essential oil or perfume. A great time to make your space sacred is while the tub is filling. Stand in the middle of the room, facing east. Close your eyes, extend your right arm out in front of you, and point your index finger. Visualize sparkly silver moon glitter coming out of your fingertip. Turn slowly around clockwise, drawing the circle, until you return to your starting point. Say, "This space is sacred and safe."

Step Two: Invoke the Goddess

Now say a prayer to acknowledge the presence of the Goddess. Your prayer might go something like this:

Goddess, I invite you to be part of my sacred ceremony

I know you are already here with me

Guide me, dear Goddess

Help me to tune into your presence

Help me to feel how special I am

Lead me to my divine nature.

Light your candle and place it in front of the mirror.

Step Three: Purification

Now step into the bathtub. If you don't have a bathtub, use a shower—you can also use the shower for the mini-version of this ceremony, just skip the bubble bath. Gently wash your skin with a facecloth and imagine all your worries and concerns, insecurities and upsets are washing right off you. Close your eyes and lie back in the bath. Don't put your head under the water—I don't want you to drown! Breathe deeply, allow your body to relax, and imagine you are in the womb of the Goddess. Feel the water soothe and comfort you. Know you are completely safe in the arms of the Goddess.

Step Four: Anoint Yourself as Goddess

After you get out of the bath, moisturize your skin with body oil. Then stand naked in front of the mirror. If you don't feel good about your body and absolutely have a hard time looking at yourself naked and feeling good, then do step five first and come back to this step. But promise me you will work up to being able to do this naked. Take it in stages if you have to: a little naked, half naked, fully naked!

Dab some perfume on your third finger and anoint the middle of your forehead. Say: "The power of the Goddess flows through me."

Now gently dab your eyelids—don't put more perfume on to do this, as you could burn your eyes. Say: "Let me see that which is not usually seen."

Then dab perfume on your earlobes and say: "Let me hear that which is not usually heard."

Touch your lips, saying: "Let me speak, Goddess, with thoughtfulness and care."

Anoint your heart. Say: "Let me feel that which is not usually felt. May my heart be an open vessel for your love, Goddess—love which is limitless and divine." Feel the love of the Goddess radiating from your heart center now.

Dab perfume on your feet and say: "May I walk this path today with beauty and with love. May you illuminate my every step."

53

Now close your eyes and take three deep breaths. Allow your body to be filled with the presence of the Goddess. Imagine that taking place now. Then open your eyes and look directly into them in the mirror. Bring your hands together into a prayer position. Say: "Thou art Goddess, (your name). I honor the Goddess in you."

Step Five: Dress Your Goddess Self

Put on your makeup and your clothes. Do your hair. Put on your jewelry—imagine it is special magic goddess amulets. Sprinkle glitter over yourself and put on fake tattoos—do all that fun goddessy girl stuff. In the second part of this book you will have guidelines for creating specific goddess looks, or glamours. You may want to look up a particular goddess for some ideas. Once you are ready, say out loud (very loud, if possible):

I am the Goddess made manifest

The power, beauty, wisdom, and intelligence

Of the Great Goddess flow through me

I will think and act like a goddess.

Step Six: Feast and Party

Now you can eat the food you have brought. Have your own little goddess celebration. Or, if you have plans for the night, you can go out and have fun. Remember to take the silver moon glitter circle (that you made when you created your sacred space) with you when you go. Just imagine it wrapping around you as protection. Throughout the day, repeat the above goddess affirmation. I like to write it on a little card and carry it in my purse to remind me to say it.

Don't forget to write about your experience in your goddess diary before you go to sleep. Make some notes about what worked and what didn't, and how you could make it better next time.

54

Goddess Workout

Rewrite the ceremony into a shorter version that you can use every day as part of your bathing routine. Use it tomorrow.

Celebrate your goddess self!

Gifts of the Inner Goddess

Your inner goddess is overflowing with gifts for you to use. She will show you how to tune into the realm of the invisible and how to awaken your spiritual senses. By listening to the messages of your inner goddess, you will learn how to receive Goddess guidance, how to accurately read people, how to practice wise judgment, and how to make good decisions.

You will become aware that you are always divinely guided, no matter what is going on in your life. On good days and bad days, happy days and sad days, calm days and angry days, the Goddess is always with you, and you can tune into divine guidance no matter how you feel.

You will start to see the universe as a magical world and look beyond apparent problems to spiritual solutions. You will clear the channels of communication between you and the Goddess. You will start receiving goddess guidance more regularly in the form of visual messages, audio messages, intuitive messages, and bodily messages. You may actually see the Goddess or your guardian angels, fairies, or animal allies.

You will notice your sensory perceptions expand; colors seem more vibrant, hearing seems clearer, and you will become more aware of the life force in everything. You will get strobe-light clarity about a situation or person that has been bothering you. Soon you will feel the presence of the invisible almost as tangibly as if you could reach out and touch it.

People sometimes think becoming more psychic requires you to be kind of a space cadet. What I have found is that it really requires you to become more grounded—to pay greater attention to detail, not less; to be more in your body; to practice wise judgment instead of trying to transcend it; to trust your own connection to the divine; and to trust yourself.

How the Goddess Can Communicate with You

The Goddess will communicate with you through your spiritual senses. Your spiritual senses are the gifts of your inner goddess. These gifts open the channels of communication between you and divinity so that you can converse with the Goddess easily and clearly.

What Are Your Spiritual Senses?

We each have four spiritual senses. These are commonly called clairvoyance, clairaudience, clairsentience, and claircognition. I call them spiritual sight, spiritual hearing, spiritual sensing, and spiritual knowing.

Just like you probably have one or two physical senses that are more dominant in you than your other senses, so it is with your spiritual senses. It is common to have one spiritual sense that is stronger in you than the others. However, you can learn to use all your spiritual senses to expand your perception of spiritual reality.

Spiritual Perception and Ordinary Perception

We perceive the world around us through our senses. Everything in the physical, manifest universe is experienced by us through our sight, sound, smell, taste, and touch. Ordinary reality is how things appear to us through our physical senses and rational mind.

Spiritual perception is the ability to perceive the spiritual reality surrounding us through our spiritual senses. The spiritual universe is there, whether we perceive it or not.

What Is the Spiritual Universe?

Everything has a spiritual double, which is their spiritual essence. The spiritual universe surrounds us. Remember when I said we are all made from the same spiritual substance? Well, the spiritual universe is what connects us all together.

There is a fifth dimension of quantum reality that exists even though most of us can't see it with our physical senses. Aborigines call this dimension the Dreamtime, Celtic people call it the Otherworld, and some people call it the astral plane —the place where all magic begins.

I like to think of the spiritual universe as being superimposed over and within our physical universe. If you can think of a computer program that works with layers, you may find it easier to understand how the spiritual universe exists. Let's say you are working with seven layers. You turn off the top layer and the bottom layer. You can still see the other five layers, but not the two that are switched off. That doesn't mean they are not there anymore—you just can't see them.

When you sharpen your spiritual senses and practice using them, you will begin to perceive the spiritual universe until you can see it as clearly as you perceive the physical universe. It's kind of like the night sky. Even though you can't see stars during the day, they are always there.

By using tools like meditation to heighten your awareness of spiritual perception, you will start to perceive spiritual reality.

Let me give you an example. A few years ago, my marriage hit a crisis. My husband was going through a deep depression. He didn't know if he wanted to be married anymore. He didn't know what he wanted to do with his life. On the surface, things looked bad. I was afraid I was going to end up a single mother raising our two sons alone. My spiritual senses told me this was not the case. They said that my husband would soon come to his senses and everything in our marriage would be fine.

When I looked at things from an ordinary perception, I felt afraid, unloved, and rejected. When I looked at things from a spiritual perspective, I understood Stephen was going through his own private turmoil right now, but I could see in the future that everything was going to be okay and our marriage would not only survive, but thrive.

Spiritual Sight

Clairvoyance is the ability to see clearly. It is how you receive visual messages from the Goddess.

With your spiritual sight, you can:

+ See auras

+ Have visions

+ See things in your dreams

+ See things in your imagination that appear out of the blue, like events unfolding in a certain way

+ See places you have never been to before or see people you have never met before—then one day you go to the place or meet the person

+ See energy around people or objects

+ See colors emanating from people or objects that give you an insight into their emotional state, like gray for depression, red for anger, green for jealousy, pink for love, or orange for joy

+ Keep seeing a certain name, phrase, or number in different places

+ See angels, fairies, or other spiritual beings, including goddesses

The Goddess can communicate with you through your spiritual sight by giving you dreams and visions and the ability to see events unfolding in a certain way in your mind. You may receive mental pictures or mental movies from her.

When my marriage was in crisis and I prayed for insight, I could see very clearly in my imagination how everything was going to turn out.

How do you know this is not just wishful thinking or fantasizing? Well, you pray about it first. You ask the Goddess to send you a picture of what you need to know, do, or how the situation will be. At first you may feel like you are making it up. After a while, as you have more experience with things turning out the way you saw them, you will trust your spiritual senses more readily. Practice makes perfect!

The Goddess will never send you frightening messages or tell you to do something that goes against your morals or your conscience. If this should ever happen (it has never happened to me), pray immediately to the Goddess to remove the negative thoughtforms from your mind and body.

59

Goddess Workout

Have you ever experienced spiritual sight? If so, write about it in your goddess journal.

Practice looking at people and see if you can see their energy.

Ask the Goddess to send you a visual message about a situation you would like information about.

Spiritual Hearing

Clairaudience is the ability to hear clearly. It is how to receive audio messages from the Goddess.

With your spiritual hearing, you can:

- Hear a voice outside your head giving you a specific message

- Hear a voice inside your head giving you a specific message

- Hear fragments of other people's conversations that seem like a direct message to you

- Hear a song on the radio that seems to be talking straight to you

- Hear a person on TV saying something that tells you exactly what you need to know

- Hear the voice of the Goddess or the angels giving you specific advice

When my marriage was in crisis, I frequently heard the Goddess and the angels giving me all kinds of messages. The angels told me they were sending me a thousand angels to take care of me and my sons. I thought this was kind of excessive, but that's what they said! They said they were sending my husband five hundred angels to take care of him. Each day they told me not to worry, that everything would turn out fine, that our marriage was not going to be over—we still had a long way to go.

I could hear my husband's spirit self talking to me, telling me to hold on, that Stephen's ordinary self was just going through a rough time and needed some space to work things out but that he loved me dearly. At nighttime, as I lay in bed, Stephen's spirit body would show up just like a guardian angel and sit down and talk to me. He would say things like, "Please be patient with me. I love you so very, very much."

During the day, Stephen's ordinary self was confused and he would vacillate between not knowing what to do and being angry and upset. It was a very emotional time. But I tried to focus on my spiritual perception of the situation and the messages I was getting instead of focusing on the surface reality.

It was two and a half months of emotional turmoil. but one evening Stephen sat down on our bed and said: "Catherine, I'm back. I am so sorry, will you forgive me?" We both cried. That was a real turning point in our marriage because Stephen has always been a great person but from that moment he changed. It wasn't like he became a totally different person but his identity expanded of what he was capable of. He gained so much certainty about himself and what he wanted for his life and for our marriage and our children.

Sometimes you have to go through the alchemical fires of hell to receive the gold.

Interestingly, about a month later I went to hear Doreen Virtue give an angel workshop near where I lived. She looked over at me in the audience at one point and said, "That woman has so many angels floating around her, it looks like she is in an aquarium filled with angels!"

I smiled to myself, thinking of what the angels had said about sending me one thousand angels to take care of things.

Often I write down the messages I hear the Goddess or the angels giving me. Sometimes, years later, I will reread what I have written and it never ceases to amaze me how accurate their advice is.

Goddess Workout

Sit down at a computer with a word-processing program open. Turn the computer screen off. Ask the Goddess a question. Pray: *"Goddess, guide my fingers on the keyboard,"* then write down what you "hear." Don't worry if you feel like you are making it up. Just do it anyway. After twenty minutes, turn the computer screen back on and read what you have written.

If you don't have a computer, try this exercise using a pen and paper and do it with your eyes closed.

You can ask a specific question to any problem or challenge you are having, too.

Spiritual Sensing

Clairsentience is the ability to feel clearly. It is how to receive messages in your body and emotions from the Goddess.

With your spiritual sense of feeling, you can:

- Experience intuition

- Experience gut feelings or hunches

- Feel other sensations in your body that seem to give you a specific message

- Sense how things will turn out

- Feel auras

- Sense another's energy without them having to utter a word

I have had several interesting experiences of spiritual sensing. One Saturday night, when I was a teen, I was driving around town and I got a sick, panicky feeling in the pit of my stomach. I knew my boyfriend, who was supposed to be home studying, was on a date with another girl. I just knew it. I could feel it—even though I had no reason to believe this was the case. I asked him later and my sense was correct. Boy, was he in big trouble!

What if you have days when your ordinary senses kick in and you can't seem to get in touch with your spiritual senses? Well, I have had plenty of days like that, too.

I have had days when I didn't feel like everything would be all right. There were days when I felt everything was just terrible. On those days, I would walk mindlessly around a park, screaming to myself, "I believe in a power much greater than myself." "I believe in divine timing." "I believe the Goddess can make a way where there is no way." I really wasn't feeling too much like I believed those things, but I kept repeating them anyway.

I would just stomp around the park in endless circles for forty-five minutes or until I was exhausted, making these statements out loud to the universe and to myself.

These were my "marching orders." I felt as if I was in spiritual military camp, training my mind to think correctly, blocking out all the thoughts of doubt and fear and impossibility that would fill my mind when I assessed the situation from an ordinary perspective.

As soon as I felt I could "power walk" no longer, I would go home and collapse into bed, envisioning the Goddess holding me and comforting me.

Goddess Workout

Pay attention to any messages your body seems to be giving you about a situation or person.

See if you can feel the energy of a room when you walk into it. Do this in restaurants, classrooms, shops, or parties.

See if you can gauge what someone's mood is before they begin talking to you.

Pay attention to your intuition. What messages is your intuition giving you today?

Spiritual Knowing

Claircognition is the ability to know clearly. It is how to receive factual messages and information from the Goddess.

When you experience spiritual knowing, you can:

+ Get facts and figures in your mind seemingly out of nowhere

+ Know where a missing object is

+ Think clearly from a spiritual perspective

+ Know the truth about a situation

+ Know when someone is lying to you

+ Instantly know something about a person or a situation without being told

Claircognition is how you know who is on the phone before it rings. Or you might meet someone and know they have had an abortion at one time in their life. You might know the answer to a question someone asks you even though you have never studied the subject matter. You might know something is going to occur—like a death, a job promotion, or a friend's betrayal before it happens.

My friend Maya was talking about one of our friends and his wife one day when she said, "soon to be ex-wife." We all stared at her, stunned. "Where did that come from?" we were wondering. The words popped out, apparently from nowhere. We had no reason to believe the marriage was in crisis. Three weeks later, we learned our friend had indeed left his wife.

....

Goddess Workout

Develop your imagination and intuition to receive goddess guidance and see the invisible realms. Use the tools from your magical toolbox on page 29 to help you. Meditation, visualization, affirmations, and prayers are wonderful tools for opening your intuition and your imagination.

Practice guessing who is on the phone when it rings.

Goddess Helpers:
How They Can Assist You

There are many different spirit beings and they all have very different purposes and abilities to help you. You are surrounded by help from the spiritual world. Call on these beings to help you regularly. These goddess helpers love to work with humans. The only condition is that you ask them first. Because of the law of free will, goddess helpers can only intervene if you ask them to, unless you are in a life-threatening situation before your time. You can also call on these beings to help your loved ones, too.

Angels

Angels are mentioned in nearly every religion. Everyone has at least one guardian angel. There are many different kinds of angels: archangels, cherubs, tiny sprite-like angels, large luminous angels. There are angels who specialize in different areas—writing angels, running angels, beauty angels, homework angels, romance angels—you name it. There are angels for every single thing!

I love working with the angels and I call on them daily for help. You can call on the angels by simply saying, "Angels, help!" The angels love to help humans—it gives them great joy and delight to do so. They wish we would call on them more often! You can call on them for help with absolutely anything, from big things to tiny things. If you cut your leg while shaving or if you are looking for a parking space or if you have a major crisis in your life, just call out to the angels.

Call on specific angels for specific needs. If you are going swimming, call on the swimming angels to come, too. If you are troubled by your looks, call on the beauty angels to help you; if you have a first date with someone, call on the romance angels. If you are in a dangerous situation or are at home by yourself and feel afraid, call on the bodyguard angels. The angels come the instant you call.

Your guardian angel is always with you and you can develop a close relationship with her (or him!) by talking to her every day. I use writing as a way to talk to my angels. I ask them a question, then write down the answer. I talk to my angels throughout the day in my mind, too, just having mental conversations with them.

I do this with the Goddess as well. Sometimes I even talk out loud to her. Knowing you are surrounded by angels is such a comforting feeling—you never feel lonely or unloved. They are so helpful, giving assistance to every area of your life.

I hope you contact your angels every single day. The magic, healing, and love they have poured into my life is amazing, and I know they want to do the same for you, too. All you need to do is ask them.

....

Goddess Workout

Close your eyes and ask your guardian angel to appear to you. Sometimes you may sense her presence rather than see her. Have a mental conversation with her about whatever is going on in your life.

Priestesses

Priestesses are beings who serve the Goddess. Many of them have lived on Earth at one time, serving the Goddess in a goddess temple. They are wise women who can counsel you with specific goddess suggestions for improving any area of your life. When you ask a priestess for guidance, it is very much like going to talk to a minister at a church. These priestesses work in the goddess temples in the spiritual universe. I see the priestesses wearing long white gowns with beautiful blue robes over them. They often wear beautiful goddess jewelry.

You can imagine going to a goddess temple where a priestess of the Goddess greets you. She will take you to a special room in the temple and sit with you. You can tell her whatever is on your mind and get divine assistance from her.

Priestesses are wonderful goddess counselors for whatever is going on in your life. They offer wise and gentle guidance. They are trained in the areas of healing and counseling, opening your spirituality, sexuality, love, relationships, and careers. They have dedicated their lives to the Goddess and exist solely to do her work and help you on your goddess path.

You can ask the Goddess to assign you your own personal priestess to help you with your goddess work. Talk to your priestess every day. She will function as a mentor and counselor to you in your goddess training. The priestess will help train you on your goddess path by giving you specific exercises and activities to do. She can help you plan ceremonies and advise you on what spiritual books, classes, or tasks you would find beneficial to do.

....

Goddess Workout

Close your eyes and do a meditation to go to a goddess temple. Visit with a priestess and have a conversation with her. Write down your experience in your goddess journal.

Fairies

Most of the fairies that I work with come from the Celtic realms. There are a lot of fairies in the Celtic tradition like Fand, the Celtic Fairy Queen of love and beauty. However, other traditions have fairies, too! Fairies love nature. They live in flowers, rivers, waterfalls, trees, and any natural setting.

Many years ago I prayed to the fairies that I would be able to see them. They sent me this information in a dream. "If you want to see us," they said, "look for us as you would look for dust particles in the sunlight. When the sun is a certain height and you see dust streaming through the light of a window, that is how you can see us, too. You will see our wings or our whole bodies." Many times since then I have caught glimpses of the fairies at certain times of the day when the light is diffused.

Fairies come in all different sizes and shapes, as do angels. There are large, human-size fairies, such as fairies from the Celtic Otherworld, and delightful, tiny fairies, such as the flower fairies or Tinkerbell.

Nature fairies are playful and will bring delight and joy into your life. Celtic fairies have all different qualities. If you want to know more about the different types of fairies and how to work with them, read *A Witches' Guide to Faery Folk* by Edain McCoy.

....

Goddess Workout

Leave some food for the fairies by a tree or a patch of flowers. They especially love bits of cake and sweet drinks.

Make a fairy mound in your backyard. This is where you dedicate a small corner to the fairies—an area of about four inches by four inches is fine. Leave tiny ribbons, bells, trinkets, and sparkly beads there for the fairies to play with. And, every so often, leave them a little food, too. They love cake! The fairies will be delighted and will reward you with much playfulness and laughter.

Power Animals

Power animals are animals that exist in the spirit world and will come to your aid when you ask them to. How can power animals help you? Well, you can call on a specific animal that is renowned for its qualities, like a lion if you want to be more regal or if you want protection, or a dolphin if you want to be more playful and trusting. Birds will help you to see things from a higher perspective, to get the overall view of a situation. You can ask a guard dog to protect you and your possessions. You can call on mythical animals, too, like dragons and unicorns.

Here's a list of some animals and their correspondences:

BAT: psychic powers, travel to other realms, clairvoyance

BEAR: protectiveness

BUTTERFLY: beauty, rejuvenation, lightheartedness, hope

CAT: perception, insightfulness, self-containment

CROW: initiation, prophecy, death or birth, strong sense of self

DEER: empowerment, leadership, responsibility, compassion

DOG: loyalty, protection, guidance, patience

DOLPHIN: fun, loyalty, empathy, kindness, joy, intuition

DRAGON: power, ferocity, independence, challenge

DRAGONFLY: magic, impulsiveness, flightiness

EAGLE: far-seeing, visionary, freedom

FOX: cunningness, wiliness, wittiness

GRYFFIN: sovereignty, protection, honor

HORSE, BLACK: wisdom, intuition, transformation

HORSE, BROWN: dependability, loyalty, courage

HORSE, WHITE: love, beauty, otherworldliness, spirituality

LION: strength, sovereignty, power, courage, pride in yourself and your tasks

OWL: wisdom, patience

SALMON: wisdom, study

SKUNK: setting boundaries, playfulness, flirtatiousness, protection

SNAKE: renewal, transformation, starting new habits

SPIDER: destiny, handiwork, creativity

SWAN: beauty, purity, grace

TOAD: protection from enemies, stalwartness

TURTLE: perseverance, determination

UNICORN: magic, inner and outer beauty, focused mind, intelligence

WOLF: intuition, protection, motherliness

Many goddesses had sacred animals that were their companions. Some goddesses were associated with different animals and could take on the shape of that animal, like Rhiannon, the horse goddess from Celtic mythology. You can call on the animal of a specific goddess, too.

Very often if you have had a beloved pet who has died, this pet will be your power animal and stay close by your side, bringing you comfort and joy. If you want to learn more about the spiritual qualities of animals and how to work with them, there are many great books and card decks available. Do a search online for animal cards and check out authors like Jamie Sams and John Matthews for their work on the magical attributes of animals.

Ancestors

Your ancestors just love to help you, as you carry their blood within you. Call on your ancestors that you know are experienced in certain areas. For example, I called on my Uncle Kere when I wanted to quit smoking, as he had quit smoking cold turkey after smoking three packs a day for many years. I call on my Grandma Sadie for help with psychic readings. I never knew her—she died before I was born—but she was the seventh daughter of a seventh daughter and used to read tea leaves. She had "the sight."

When I am in a difficult situation or I feel trouble looming, I call on my Celtic ancestors and my Maori ones. I imagine them all standing beside me, behind me, and in front of me, protecting me and guiding me.

Sometimes I call on an ancestor of mine who lived in the sixteenth century and was burned at the stake in Scotland for witchcraft.

....

Goddess Workout

Which ancestors of yours would you like to call on and why?

Meditation to Open Your Spiritual Centers

Read or record this first.

Lie down, close your eyes. Feel your body becoming relaxed. Take a deep breath in and hold it for four seconds, then exhale. Do this three times.

You are now becoming more and more relaxed. Deeper and deeper, you feel your consciousness slip into a wonderful, deep slumber where you don't need to worry about anything. You feel all the tension leaving your body. You feel your body relaxing and opening up like a flower in the sunshine.

You begin to notice your surroundings and find you are in a grassy meadow filled with sweet-smelling flowers of all different colors. Just nearby there is a beautiful waterfall and you see sparkles of pink and green and yellow and all the colors of a rainbow radiating from the waterfall. There are woodland creatures that hover nearby, squirrels and bunny rabbits, and you even catch a glimpse of a white unicorn in the distance, coming toward you, and you notice a baby dragon sunbathing on a rock.

Soon you see a group of priestesses walking serenely toward you. They form a circle around your body, like a flock of angels. They are smiling. They wear beautiful, long, blue silk gowns and on their wrists and around their necks are the most beautiful pieces of goddess jewelry you have ever seen.

They ask your permission to work on your body, healing it and regenerating it while you relax. You willingly agree—you feel so comforted, nurtured, and loved in their presence. You know they would never do anything to harm you or lead you astray.

The priestesses work deftly, running their hands all over your body, clearing away any old emotional wounds and scars. They take away all regrets from the present and the past, all resentments, all heartaches and disappointments, and all self-punishment in the form of thinking mean things about yourself, saying mean things to yourself, and allowing others to say mean things to you.

They take away all hurts from your heart center in the forms of unrequited love, betrayal, disappointment, heartbreaks, lack of self-love, and anything that has hurt your heart in any way.

You feel your body becoming lighter and lighter, and it feels so good to be free and open. Next the priestesses lay their hands on you. One of them stands at the top of your head and places her hands on your forehead, sending purple light throughout your body. You feel a jolt of energy rush through you, opening the top of your head.

Now another priestess lays her hands on your brow, and you feel a jolt of indigo energy opening up your third-eye area. This is the place where you receive psychic visions.

Another priestess places her hands gently over your ears and you feel a warm liquid flowing through them, clearing them out. The priestess pours loving energy into your ears to amplify the sound of the Goddess communicating with you.

Now a priestess gently places her palms on your throat and tells you this is your center of spiritual communication. You see a beautiful blue light radiating around your throat. The priestess says, "May you always speak with the words of the Goddess, may you always see the beauty of the Goddess, and may you always hear the voice of the Goddess."

The next priestess places her warm palms firmly on your heart region, and you see a beautiful pink light shot with flickers of green emanating from her hands and filling your heart and your entire upper torso. The light feels like liquid honey; it is so warm and nourishing. You allow your heart center to open wider and wider, knowing, as you do so, that you will receive so much love and joy from the Goddess and other people, and you in turn will give out so much love and joy.

Then a priestess lays her hands on your belly, and you feel your whole lower torso filling with red, orange, and yellow energy. This energy is warm and vibrant, filling you like the sun on a midsummer's day. You see the colors all swirling around inside you and emanating from you. The priestess tells you that this energy will give you strength, vitality, determination, focus, and amazing self-confidence. It will ignite the fires of your creative centers and keep them burning brightly so you will be a beacon of love and beauty and confidence for all who see you.

Finally a priestess holds your feet and sends loving energy throughout your body, explaining to you that with her help you will be able to manifest all your spiritual gifts in the material world. She will guide your feet to walk the ways of the Goddess in this lifetime.

Now you feel so vibrant and healthy and power-full. You feel as if you could achieve anything. You see all the colors the priestesses have poured into you circling throughout your body like a beautiful, magnificent rainbow. This, the priestesses tell you, is your very own inner holy spirit. Your inner holy spirit is forever eternally connected to the spirit of the Goddess; her divine love, wisdom, joy, beauty, and guidance are yours to enjoy right now.

You thank the priestesses and they smile and say they are always with you, watching out for you. Then you feel your body start to come back to the present time, the present room, and your consciousness is aware of all that is going on around you. Slowly, slowly, you come back to where you are lying. When you are ready, open your eyes.

Goddess Workout

Write about your meditation experience in your goddess journal.

Ways to Enhance Your Spiritual Senses

Your spiritual senses thrive on many kinds of soul food; you can feed your spiritual senses with this nourishment so they become clearer, stronger, and more finely attuned. Here are some things you can surround yourself with that will feed your spiritual senses:

- Eating fresh fruits, especially melons and pineapple

- Bells

- Harp music

- Walking in nature

- Fresh flowers

- Any beautiful instrumental music

- Candles

- Crystals

- Meditation

- Deep prayer

- Aromatherapy oils

- Tarot cards or visual pictures that act as a doorway into the spiritual realm when you gaze on them for a while

- Angel or goddess figurines or statues

- Silk scarves

Goddess Workout

Set aside an hour one evening this week, preferably when the sun has gone down. In your bedroom, create a sacred space to honor your spiritual senses. Choose a few things off the above list and make your bedroom into a mini-goddess temple so you can sit and pray with the Goddess while all your spiritual senses are being enhanced.

Practicing Wise Judgment

One of the most useful gifts of the inner goddess is the gift of discernment. This is the ability to practice wise judgment. What is wise judgment? This is not passing judgment on others for their actions or their personalities, but rather being able to discern if a person or situation is healthy for you. How can you tell? By tuning in to your intuition and paying attention to how you feel after you have spent time with a certain person. If you continually feel drained or belittled after being around someone, then this is a good sign that this person is not right for you.

Sometimes when you meet someone you will get a message in your body or a sense that this person will only bring you trouble. Pay attention to your first impressions of someone. Very often when you get a strong first impression, you are picking up the energy of that person. Trust these impressions, as they are seldom incorrect.

If you have someone in your life who makes you feel bad about yourself, turn the relationship over to the Goddess and ask her for help to remove this person from your life or to help you develop the skills and resources to stand up for yourself.

75

Goddess Workout

Practice using wise judgment this week. Notice which friends make you feel good about yourself and which ones seem to tease you or pick on you or drain you a lot. Ask the Goddess for help with these relationships.

*Let your inner
goddess guide you*

Conjuring Your Destiny

Would you like to have more control over where you are going physically, mentally, and emotionally? Destiny is the power that determines the course of events. When it comes to your own life, you have a great deal of power in determining how things turn out. When you ask the Goddess for help, you have unlimited access to the greatest power of all.

Sometimes events may happen where it seems as if you have no control: you lose a job, your science teacher picks on you, you are in an accident, your boyfriend dumps you, your best friend says mean things about you behind your back. . . . You may not be able to stop any of these situations from happening, but you can always control your reactions and how you go about picking up the pieces. You can always ask the Goddess for help, too.

To take charge of your destiny, you need to have a magical vision of what you want your life to be about. You need to set goals to help you, and you need to think about what kind of person you want to be. You need to use language, thoughts, and actions to support your vision, and you need to call on the Goddess and her helpers for support and guidance. By doing this, you will learn how to make your dreams a reality.

The Amazing, Incredible Power of the Goddess

There are three qualities often assigned to describe the power of divinity. These are omniscience, omnipresence, and omnipotence. Let's talk about omnipotence first.

The Goddess Is Omnipotent (All-Powerful)

Think about this statement for a moment. The Goddess is all-powerful. What does this mean? Close your eyes for a moment and imagine all the power of the universe—and more—at your fingertips. How would you use it? What would you do? *Omnipotence* means "all power." Not just a *little* power or a *lot* of power but *all* power. Divine power is so great that it manifested the universe and everything in it. It is so great that it holds the planets in their perfect places in our galaxy, and it holds and supports you just as easily and effortlessly.

The Goddess is so powerful that she can do anything. Absolutely anything. When you rely on the power of the Goddess, amazing things will happen and you will always be divinely guided and divinely protected.

So let's think a little bit more about the immense power of the Goddess. Think about the power you see around you. There is the power of electricity, which causes our houses to be warm, our hair dryers to work, and our computers to function. There is the power generated by airplanes effortlessly moving millions of people from one country to another at any given moment. There is the power of the sun, warming our bodies and providing food for us to eat. There are many different types of power, like nuclear power, solar power, and hydropower, and they are all different aspects of the divine power of the Goddess.

78

....
Goddess Workout

Write down five different types of power you can think of right now.

Write down what these various powers are capable of doing: sending people to the moon, blowing up the entire planet ten times over, etc.

Since the Goddess is all-powerful, think about how much more powerful she is than all these various powers put together. What a lot of power that is, and you have access to it right now. There is never a problem or dilemma facing you that the Goddess can't help you resolve.

The Goddess Is Omniscient (All-Knowing)

The Goddess knows everything! She is divine wisdom, divine knowledge, and divine understanding. She is the keeper of the Akashic Records, where all the events of all time—past, present, and future—are recorded and stored. There is not one single problem in the whole entire universe that the Goddess does not know the answer to. She knows how to heal any situation, she knows the cure for every disease, and she knows the resolution to any problem.

When you are facing a tough decision or can't find something that is lost, the Goddess knows the answer to that, too. She just knows everything. Pretty cool, huh? For any question or problem you might have, the Goddess always knows the absolute right thing to do for it.

The Goddess Is Omnipresent (All-Present)

The Goddess is everywhere. There is not a single place where she does not reside. She is with you right now. She is in the stars, the moon, and the sun. She is in your cells, your bones, and your blood. She is in the atoms and the molecules that make up the material world. She is in the ether and the atmosphere that make up the spiritual world. Think of her like a great big cloud that envelops everything. She is always with you. When you are in your deepest, darkest moment, when you are having the time of your life, and when you are just chilling, the Goddess is always there. There is never a problem or situation facing you where you must face it alone. Always, always the Goddess is there to help you, guide you, and protect you.

Use Your Goddess Power

Claim your goddess power and use your goddess power every day!

Write Down What You Want

The first step to solving problems or making your dreams come true is to write down on a piece of paper what you want. If you don't know yet what you want, don't worry—begin with writing what you *don't* want. So before we go any further, grab a cup of hot chocolate, your goddess journal, and a pen, and get comfortable.

Begin to write with the words *I want* or *I don't want*. Write as fast as you can until you fill up three to five pages. This exercise will take you about an hour. Don't think too much about what you are writing. Just get the words on the paper and don't worry about spelling or grammar—you are not going to be graded for this paper! Write down whatever comes to you. You may find yourself writing things like *I want a wonderful boyfriend who treats me like a princess but I can't ever have that because I'm not pretty enough.* Or you may find yourself writing *I don't know what I want. I don't know what I want. I hate my life. Nothing good ever happens to me. It's not fair. I wish I had a life like Jessica's.* . . . You may find yourself writing *I want to be the best long-distance runner in school but that is impossible because . . .* Just keep writing; write down as much as you can about what you want in every area of your life. Use the following questions as guidelines.

WHAT DO YOU WANT YOUR LIFE TO BE LIKE?

Write as much as you can about the kind of life you would like to be living. What kind of bedroom would you like to have? What kinds of friends would you like in your life? What kinds of jobs do you dream about? What activities would you like to try for fun? Are there any sports or hobbies or new skills you would like to learn? Make it as fanciful and as fun as you can. Don't worry whether it is practical or not, or whether you can believe it will actually happen. Just play make-believe and write about what you would like to be like if you had unlimited resources like money, talent, great looks, physical skills, and anything you needed to make your dreams come true.

Remember, you can do anything with the power of the Goddess. There is absolutely *no* thing you cannot do! Don't worry about how you are going to make your dreams come true. Let the Goddess and her helpers take care of that. Your job is to come up with exactly what it is that you want. Nothing is too grandiose, too expansive, too impractical, too difficult, or too impossible for the Goddess to help you attain. Your job is *what*, her job is *how*. So make your dreams as magical, as fantastical, and as powerful as you can. Dream big. Just ensure that what you want comes from your heart, not what you think you should have or be.

WHAT DO YOU WANT YOURSELF TO BE LIKE?

What kind of personality would you like to have? How would you like to feel every single day? What kinds of emotions do you want to experience on a regular basis? What do you want to look like? What kind of health habits would you like to have? How do you want your body to feel? What do you want your body to be capable of doing? What about your mind—what would you like your mind to be able to achieve? What about your self-talk—what kinds of things would you like to believe about yourself? What kinds of qualities would you like to have?

WHAT DO YOU WANT TO HAVE IN YOUR LIFE?

Okay, this is where we get into the material realm—or what you might consider materialistic. Some people think this is not very spiritual but I think the Goddess likes stuff. As you read earlier, the Goddess sure creates a lot of stuff, like zillions of snowflakes and billions of flowers, so she obviously has a keen eye for beauty and likes to surround herself with a multitude of beautiful things.

What about you? What would you like to surround yourself with? What kinds of things would you like to own? A pretty new spring dress, maybe, or a brand-new mountain bike or a great stereo? Go for it; write down things that you would really like to have if you could have anything you wanted.

What about nonmaterial things that you would like to have in your life, like a nice boyfriend, for example, or some close friends, or a good relationship with your mother? Here is where you write all those things down, too. Write about the kinds of relationships you want, write about how you want to feel in those relationships, and write about how you would like to be treated in those relationships. If it is a boyfriend you want, write down what he looks like as well as the qualities you want him to have. Write about what kind of clothes he wears, what his values are, and what kinds of activities he is into.

WHAT DON'T YOU WANT IN YOUR LIFE?

Write about all the things you wish were not in your life. If you have bad habits that you want to be rid of, write those down, too. *I don't want to be a smoker. I don't want to be friends with Aleisha anymore—she is mean. I don't want to feel stupid. I don't want to overeat. I don't want to feel miserable when I wake up in the morning. I don't want to be scared of other people. I don't want to care what other people think about me. I want people to like me. I want someone to tell me I am beautiful . . .* You get the idea. Just go for it, have fun with it.

Once you have made your lists, grab a highlighter and highlight any negatives you have written down—all the "don't wants." When you have finished highlighting all your pages, grab a separate piece of paper and turn the "don't wants" into "do wants." For example, say you wrote *I don't want to feel miserable anymore.* Write the opposite—*I want to feel happy today.* Go through each and every negative until you have written a positive that you feel happy with.

Make Your Own "Dreams Come True" Meditation Tape

Get a blank cassette or CD and start recording yourself reading your dreams aloud. Put everything into the present tense, using your positive language. Instead of saying "I want" as a preface before all the things you want, though, change it to "I see myself having" or "I see myself feeling." So you might be saying something like, "I see myself healthy, slim, and flexible. I see myself taking gym classes and eating healthy foods that I enjoy," according to the dreams on your pages. Other examples are: "I see myself having a great boyfriend who wears Doc Martens and listens to cool music and loves hanging out at the mall and I see him totally digging me and telling me I am great." Or "I see myself having a lot of confidence and walking through school holding my head up high and feeling good about myself. I see myself feeling the power of the Goddess flowing through me and I see myself surrounded by a circle of loving angels every moment of every day, protecting me and giving me love and strength."

After you have recorded all the things you see yourself having and being, take some time to record yourself seeing yourself taking actions to make your dreams come true. This is a very important step because actions are what will help manifest your dreams into the material world from the spiritual world. You can set your dreams up on the astral levels but unless you take actions in the physical world it may take awhile for them to manifest! So say something like, "I see myself taking actions every day to make my dreams come true." If you can think of specific actions to take, record yourself seeing yourself doing those, too.

The final step to making your meditation tape is to add: "I see the Goddess and her helpers helping me every single moment of every single day. I know the Goddess is all-powerful and all-intelligent and she will lead me to the right actions that I need to take and provide all the details to make my dreams come true. All I need to do is do what I can and let her take care of the rest. I know my angels are always guiding me and always protecting me. I listen openly to what they have to say." This reminds you that the Goddess is always helping you, and you are using the immense power of the divine universe to make your dreams come true. You don't have to rely solely on your own resources. Plus it sends a message to the

Goddess and the universe that you are ready to receive. Just like putting in your order at Pizza Hut, the universe doesn't know exactly what to deliver until you ask for it.

Listen to this tape every single night for six months before you go to sleep. Listen to it again in the morning if you want. It is very important to listen to this tape regularly because you are setting your dreams up in the spiritual world and reprogramming your mind to focus on what you *do* want. The more energy you put into something, the more power it has. This is an important magical principle: Focus on what you do want, not on what you don't want. Whatever we pay attention to grows—that is the law of the universe. Whatever you stop paying attention to fades away and eventually dies. You can try this principle with anything in your life.

Make a Magic Wish Box

Now gather all your pieces of paper because we are going to make a wish box. What you need is a box, like a shoebox or jewelry box. It doesn't have to be fancy. Hold the pieces of paper in your hands and say:

Dear Goddess

I place these dreams into your hands

I know with your power within me I can do anything and have anything

Help me now to make my dreams come true

Lead me toward the people, places, and resources that will help me

Guide me every step of the way

Send me angels to help make my dreams come true

With much love, your daughter.

I now expect your help and will look for signs of it showing up every day

And so it is!

You can decorate the outside of your wish box, if you want, with pretty paints or stickers. Put it away somewhere, like at the top of your closet or under your bed, and leave it there for at least six months, or even a year. Then pull it out and read all your wishes and put a check beside the ones that came true and the ones that are coming true, and note if any didn't. I believe you will be pretty amazed at the outcome of this exercise.

The Importance of Self-Responsibility and Accountability

Remember when I said earlier that blame, self-pity, and envy will keep you stuck? Well, they will. You are in charge of your life. No one else is. When you constantly blame other people for your misfortune or feel sorry for yourself about the state your life is in and what you have or don't have, you give your power away. Yes, sometimes people do hurtful things that you don't deserve. And yes, sometimes disappointments happen or accidents happen.

However, you can always take responsibility for yourself and decide what you want to do with the mess. If you are unsure what to do, pray to the Goddess for help. Call on the angels for extra help, too. Sometimes horrible things happen over which you have no control, where you may feel terribly sorry for yourself—like if you are being sexually abused or are in an accident that causes you permanent physical disabilities. I'm not saying these things are fair and in such cases you may need to go through a time of grieving where you feel terribly sorry for yourself. You may find you feel helpless and powerless and don't know what to do to take charge of the situation. You may even find you don't have the energy to even *want* to do something about the situation. If you are in such a situation, immediately pray to the Goddess to intervene. Just say, *"Goddess, help!"* She will send extra help straightaway.

Rather than praying for your problems to go away, try praying for the skills and resources to deal with them. Everybody suffers setbacks and disappointments and sometimes tragedy. When you feel overwhelmed by the events in your life, ask the Goddess to help you develop the skills and courage to take guided action.

Once I was in a situation where my boyfriend, whom I loved dearly, slept with another girl. I had to make some hard decisions about whether I wanted to stay in the relationship. I decided to stay for various reasons—too long to go into here! But for some time I wished the whole situation had never happened. I felt stuck because I couldn't undo the past; what had happened had happened, and no amount of my wishing it hadn't was going to make it *not* have happened. Finally I realized it was more productive to wish for the strength and skills to deal with it and move forward.

I asked the Goddess why we go through hard times, and this is what she said:

"Problems and difficulties are not to be feared but to be faced—head-on. They are gifts that initiate you into a different person, a wiser person, a more discerning person. They give you greater empathy, greater compassion, and deeper love. It is not the problem or difficulty that undermines you, but the way that you tackle it."

Affirmations for Using Your Goddess Power

- I am powered by the Goddess.

- My dreams are fueled by the Goddess.

- The Goddess is providing me with everything I need right now.

- The Goddess can do anything.

- The Goddess is helping me with this.

- It is in the Goddess's hands.

- I am a goddess-in-training.

- The power of the Goddess is within me.

- The Goddess loves and protects me.

- The Goddess is guiding me right now.

- Good things are happening to me today.

- My life is filled with magic.

- All things are possible to the Goddess.

- The Goddess can make all things new again.

Energy Drainers

Where does your energy go in ways that don't serve you or your vision? Energy drainers waste your time so you don't have time to accomplish your dreams. By noticing what your energy drainers are, you can begin to take steps to eliminate them. Ask the Goddess for help when you notice something that wastes your time. Energy drainers take away from your dreams and lead you nowhere.

What bad habits do you have? Do you smoke cigarettes or watch too much TV? Do you spend too much time exercising or are you a couch potato? This week, pay attention to the way you spend your time. What you learn may surprise you. Once you know where your time goes, you can see if your activities are truly things you want to put so much time into or if there are some areas you can cut back in and make things that are more important to you a priority.

The following is a list of some common energy drainers. See if you can come up with some more of your own.

Overeating or Obsessing About Your Weight

Overeating and obsessing about your weight takes up a lot of time. I know because when I was a teenager I did a lot of it! I could spend all day thinking about how I was "too fat." I could spend hours talking about diets with friends. When I overate, it made me feel disgusted with myself and made me too tired to do anything. Overeating puts a lot of stress on your digestive system, which makes you sleepy. If you have problems with overeating, look in the chapter on Gaia, the earth goddess, because we will discuss ways to deal with it. If you have problems with anorexia, look up the chapter on La Llorona for ways to nourish your starving spirit. In the meantime, give your problems to the Goddess and ask for help.

Saying or Thinking "My Life Will Be Perfect When . . ."

This is a great delay tactic. It doesn't really matter what the "when" is. It may be my life will be perfect when I have a boyfriend, my life will be perfect when I weigh 110 pounds, or my life will be perfect when I have tons of money. Actually, your life will be just the same as it is now! Don't use dreaming about the perfect future as a way of putting off your own good now. Take steps to make your life perfect today.

Alcohol or Drug Usage

Alcohol is a depressant and it will make you depressed. It depresses your energy, it depresses your emotional body, and it depresses your physical body. Also, it depresses your spiritual body, so you may find it harder to access your spiritual senses. Alcohol just numbs you. And it is the same with drugs. None of these substances serve you any constructive purpose, so there is not much point in doing them. If you have an addiction, ask the Goddess to take away your craving and seek professional help. Ask the Goddess to lead you to the perfect place for you to get help. She will.

Procrastination

Do you often find yourself procrastinating from something you want to do? You really want to lose weight but you put off exercising or eating healthy. You have an important paper due but you leave it to the last minute to do, and then start panicking about it. You want to try out for the cheerleading team but put off learning the skills. Procrastination is really just a form of fear. The task may seem too big or you may feel afraid that you don't really have the necessary skills to carry it out. When you find yourself procrastinating, pray to the Goddess for help. She will nudge you in the right direction. Sit down and break up the task into little tasks if it seems like a big job. Then do the first task on your list.

Vampire People

These are the people who suck your energy from you. I think of them as human vacuum cleaners. They take everything you have to give without giving anything in return. These may be friends who always have a problem and call you to talk about it for hours, using up your valuable time. They may be people who are always down and want you to fix things for them, or people who put their needs before yours and expect you to put everything aside to help them. Sometimes these are just people who want you to go hang out and do something mindless because they are bored. There is nothing wrong with a little mindless activity or helping a true friend in need. However, the difference between these people and true friends is that for the majority of the time you are around them, you feel tired, lethargic, or depressed after you have been with them. They are thriving on your energy!

Once I had a boyfriend who was constantly complaining that nothing was ever going right in his life. A lot of it was self-inflicted by his own choices, although I didn't know that at the time. He never had any money—he spent it all on alcohol. Everyone was against him, he moaned. He didn't know what to do with his life, he hated his friends, he hated where he lived, he hated his job, he hated his life, blah, blah, blah. . . . I would spend hours cheering him up, being his number-one supporter, coming up with creative solutions to his miserable problems.

After a while, I noticed that whenever I got home from a date with him, I was tired. It didn't matter what time of the day it was, he would feel great and I would feel exhausted. I'd have to go to bed for a couple of hours and take a nap. He was using all my energy up and I was letting him! Now I am careful not to have friends like that. I choose to put my energy into living my life and building my dreams instead of putting energy into people who, for whatever reason, choose to stay stuck. Some people just like a lot of drama and chaos in their lives!

If you have friends who drain you, ask the Goddess to help remove them from your life. They will find someone else to drain instead!

Long, Long Telephone Calls

When I was a teenager, I loved talking on the telephone. As soon as I got home from school, I would call my friends (whom I had just seen) and spend hours talking to them, one friend after another. Talking to friends on the phone is an important aspect of being a teen. Just watch the amount of time you spend doing it. Try getting off the phone sooner than you usually would, and use the extra time to do a baby task toward your dream.

Media Addictions

These include e-mail, reading magazines, hanging out at the mall, watching endless TV, playing Gameboy or Sega, or even reading tons of books all day long. There is nothing wrong with these things in moderation, but you can end up using hours and hours a day on these things if you don't pay attention. Then your dreams get pushed aside. Make sure you balance the amount of time you spend in media recreation so you have time to pursue your dreams, too.

Remember, the way you spend your time is your investment for your future. What you are doing today is determining where you will be tomorrow.

....

Goddess Workout

Make a map of your personal "wasteland," the Celtic land where everything stagnates and rots.

In Celtic mythology, the wasteland is the place where nothing grows. Everything is dead and barren. It is a desolate, depressing place—not like a desert, where there is life, but more like a waste site, filled with rotting trash, broken dreams, and polluted waters.

On a piece of paper, draw a picture of your personal wasteland; draw the activities or people who drain you. Draw the habits that harm you. Keep this picture as a reminder of the things that make your life a wasteland.

Energy Enhancers

How can you invest your energy in activities and people that support your vision? The energy enhancers are the things that lead you toward your dreams. Look for ways in your life that you can increase them.

Once you have a clear vision of what your dreams are, you can start taking steps to make them come true. Every day, do at least one thing toward your dream. When you wake up in the morning, ask the Goddess what one thing you can do today toward your dream. She will lead you to all the resources you need. It doesn't matter if the step you take is a big step or a little step. Sometimes all you may need to do is call a certain person or buy a certain book. The Goddess may advise you to spend an hour working on your dream.

Each morning before you begin your day, write down in your goddess journal the question "What one thing can I do today toward my dream, Goddess?" Then write down whatever you hear her saying or feel compelled to write. Write quickly, without editing. Write down whatever comes to mind, no matter how silly it may sound. Now you have a concrete activity that you can do that will help your dreams to manifest. If the answer you get seems too difficult for you to do, pray to the Goddess for help to carry it out.

Surround yourself with people who encourage your dreams—people who think positively and live positively, people who say, "Yes, you can do that, I know you can." Surround yourself with friends who are working toward making their dreams come true, too. If you don't have any friends like that, ask the Goddess to send you one. Ask her for a mentor. Sometimes you will have unseen mentors as well as seen ones. Unseen mentors are people who inspire you even though you don't know them. They may be celebrities or people who have achieved something you want to achieve. They may be people who are dead. You can call on them mentally for help, too. You can use their successes as encouragement and inspiration for achieving your own.

When I was a teenager, my unseen mentor was Leslie Kenton, who writes books on health and beauty and spirituality. As soon as I read her book *The Joy of*

Beauty, I was inspired to be like her. I decided right then that one day I would write books that would help people and give workshops and travel around the world speaking. Leslie's work provided me with a vision of what I wanted to do with my life. Of course it wasn't always easy sailing; I had lots of doubts and fears of not being good enough along the way, and lots of rejections, too.

Each day, ask yourself if the activity you are currently engaged in is moving you closer to your dream or taking you further away from it. Time is an investment; are you investing your time wisely into creating the kind of life you want, or are you investing your time into things that serve you no real purpose? Look for ways that you can cut down the areas where you waste time and increase the amounts of time spent in pursuit of your dreams.

92

Goddess Workout

Make a map of your "land of plenty," the Celtic land where everything grows abundantly. In the land of plenty, there is an abundance of everything: delicious foods, beautiful flowers, happy people. It is an enchanted, magical place where you can have whatever you want in abundance.

On a piece of paper, draw your own land of plenty and use it as a map to inspire you.

Be number one in your own world; learn to make yourself and your dreams a priority

Meditation to Invoke Your Goddess Power

Stand up straight, feet about a foot apart, knees slightly bent. Keep your back straight, head held up high, and your arms loosely by your sides.

Now close your eyes.

Breathe in deeply and relax.

See about two feet in front of yourself, in your imagination, your goddess self.

This is the "you" that you want to be in your wildest dreams.

See this "you" as a goddess, with all the qualities you would like to embody.

See her confident, radiant, divine.

Spend five minutes seeing yourself exactly how you would like to be, standing in front of you, as if observing another person.

Now, reach forward with your arms outstretched. Put your hands on the shoulders of this imaginary astral future "you." Pick her up slowly above your head until your arms are stretched up high. Now pull her slowly down over your head, as if you were putting on a fitted gown. Pull her down over your arms, through your torso, down your legs, all the way to your toes.

Stand up straight once more and feel yourself as this future "you," embodying all the qualities you have wanted to embody.

How do you feel?

Go forth into your day with confidence. Say: "I, (your name), am a living embodiment of the Goddess. I carry the wisdom, the power, and the strength of the Goddess with me and within me."

This meditation is based on one I learned from Reverend Patrick Pollard, whom I gratefully acknowledge.

....

Goddess Workout

Write the answers to these two questions in your goddess journal. Take about an hour to do this exercise. Make yourself a cup of hot chocolate and listen to some pretty music while you write.

What kind of life would you like to be living a year from now?

What daily actions can you take to make your dreams come true?

....

R emember, the Goddess

is always with you—

call on her for help

and make every day

a goddess day!

....

Good Morning Ceremony to Start the Day

After you have had your morning wash and are fully dressed, perform this ceremony to call upon the goddesses from the sacred circle. Stand with your eyes closed and face east; breathe deeply. Imagine the morning sun rising before you. In front of you, you see the Air Goddess, a woman with hair the color of sunshine, dressed in a flowing yellow gown. You ask her to bless your plans and dreams for today with her divine light and wisdom. Ask her to inspire your mind with creative ideas, sharpen your intellect, and give you the power of a sharp wit and quick tongue. Pray: "Bless my words, O Mother, that all that may spring forth from my lips blesses your holy name. Bless my thoughts, O Mother, that all that my mind dwells upon is aligned with my vision for my life."

Now turn and face the south. Before you stands the Fire Goddess, a woman with flaming red hair and intense, penetrating eyes. She is passionate and lively. You ask her blessings for this day that everything you undertake will be done with her enthusiasm and passion. Ask for her help to actively bring your dreams alive. Pray: "Bless my actions, O Mother, that all that I do may bless your holy name. Give me strength, power, and confidence on this day."

Next, turn and face the west. Before you stands the Water Goddess. She has luminous blue eyes and wears a floating blue gown shimmering with the colors of the sea. You ask her to bless your dreams and plans for the day with her overflowing love. Ask her to guide your emotions and your moods so that all that you feel may be a blessing to her. Pray: "Guide me today, O Mother, and may my heart dwell upon the ocean of your endless love. May my plans and dreams be infused with love upon this day so all that I feel blesses your holy name."

Turn to the north. Before you stands the Earth Goddess. She is wearing a long green velvet gown and has eyes the color of rich, fertile soil. Adorning her dress are flowers and fruits. Her body is tall and willowy, like an ancient tree. You ask her to help you manifest your dreams and plans on this day. Pray: "May the beauty of this day unfold before me. May my dreams and visions be grounded and manifest in the solid foundation of your love, O Bountiful Mother."

Now you have completed the circle. Turn once more to the east and say: "Goddess before me, Goddess behind me, Goddess at my right, Goddess at my left, Goddess above me and Goddess below me. I go forth this day with the power of the Goddess!"

See the Goddess helping you throughout the day.

Good Night Ceremony to End the Day

Now it is time to end the day with the sacred circle of goddesses. Start first in the north and, with your eyes closed, see the Earth Goddess before you. Say: "I give thanks for this day, O Mother. I place today and all that I manifested in your hands. Guard my dreams and visions while I sleep."

Turn to the west and see the Water Goddess. Say: "I place all my relationships in your hands, O Mother. Guard my friends and family while I sleep. Cleanse my heart with your gentle waters so I may awaken refreshed in the morning."

Next turn to the south and see the Fire Goddess. Say: "I put all my deeds of today in your hands, O Mother. I give you all my difficulties, too, to take care of for me. Cleanse and heal my body. Give me sweet dreams that I may awaken joyous in the morning."

Now it is to the east and the Air Goddess that you turn. Say: "O Mother, cleanse and heal my mind that all my thoughts may be purified and aligned with your perfect spirit during the night. Send your gentle winds to purify every cell in my body as I sleep."

When you lie down in your bed to go to sleep, imagine all four goddesses standing in a circle around you, with their helpers guarding you, healing you, and replenishing and protecting you with their sacred magic during the night. Know that you are a beloved daughter of the Goddess and that she is guiding and protecting you right now.

Use your goddess power!

SECTION TWO

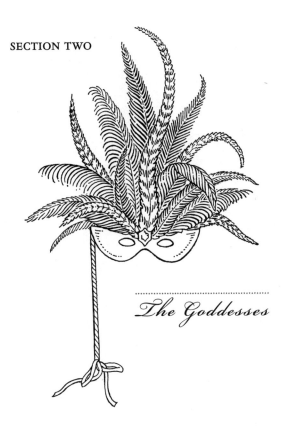

The Goddesses

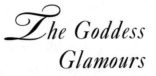

The Goddess Glamours

In this section you will meet fifteen different goddesses from different cultures around the world. Some of them, like Kuan Yin and Mary, are still worshipped today. Some of them, like Gaia and Aphrodite, were worshipped many years ago by tons of people, and had temples built in their honor. Some of them, like Queen Boadicea and Bridget, were women who actually lived.

Use these chapters as guidelines to create your own embodiment of the Goddess. You may feel drawn to work with a particular goddess whose physical representation is similar to yours, or you may feel drawn to work with one who has qualities you would like to emulate. You may feel an affinity with a goddess from your culture or ancestry, or you may have a current situation that one of the goddesses would be best suited for dealing with.

Each chapter has a story about that goddess, the challenges she faced, and how she overcame them. At the end of each chapter is a goddess glamour for that goddess, so you can learn how to manifest her in the physical realm through your body.

Working with the goddesses is very much a copartnership. When you do a glamour, you embody the spiritual essence of the goddess, which brings us to the next question . . .

What Is a Glamour?

A glamour is an enchantment that makes you appear a certain way to those who see you. You can use beauty magic to be more glamorous, no matter what you look like. According to the dictionary, "glamour" is the quality of being fascinatingly attractive, alluring, and full of excitement, adventure, and unusual activity. Nowhere in the dictionary does it say anything about you needing to have a perfect nose, weigh 120 pounds, or be six feet tall to be glamorous!

An older meaning of "glamour" is a spell, magic, or enchantment—and that's the meaning we are talking about here. A good example of a glamour is in the story of Cinderella when her fairy godmother transforms Cinderella from scullery maid to a beautiful princess for the ball. Cinderella appears as a beautiful princess to all who see her until the clock strikes midnight and the glamour fades.

Women have been using beauty magic since time began. When Cleopatra wanted to attract Mark Antony, she used beauty magic to appear as Aphrodite, the goddess of love and beauty. Women in India often dress themselves up to appear as their favorite goddess, and you can, too. All you need to do is throw a glamour.

How to Throw a Glamour

Throwing a glamour is very much like preparing for a part in a play. You invoke the qualities of a particular goddess you want to project, and use costume and makeup to dress up as that goddess, just like an actress would to make a character she is playing more believable.

Throwing a glamour is fun. People often throw glamours unconsciously before important events. When you see a cute guy and try to present your best side, when you get dressed up for the prom, when you go for a job interview and want to project your good qualities—all these are glamours.

Sometimes people unknowingly throw negative glamours, too, like when you think negative stuff about yourself. When you put yourself down or criticize your appearance, you are unwittingly weaving a web of negativity around yourself.

Whenever jealousy, self-hate, or self-pity consume you, you aren't allowing your true beauty to shine forth. The way to turn this negativity around is to change your thinking and start believing in yourself. You can use a little goddess power to help, too.

To throw a glamour, all you need to do is:

1. Use your imagination.

2. Create a costume.

3. Invoke your goddess power.

4. Use makeup, jewelry, and perfume for magical props.

5. Call on a goddess to help you and let her energy infuse you and radiate out from you.

So let's get going and meet the goddesses!

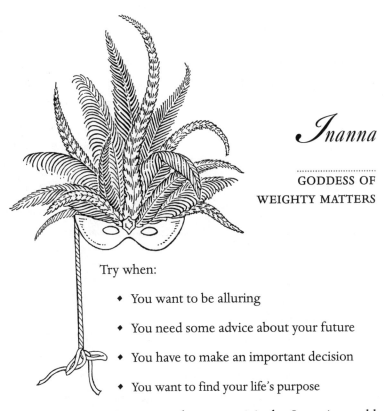

Inanna

GODDESS OF
WEIGHTY MATTERS

Try when:

+ You want to be alluring

+ You need some advice about your future

+ You have to make an important decision

+ You want to find your life's purpose

Inanna (pronounced *ee-naa-naa*) is the Sumerian goddess of the sun, moon, and stars. She is the goddess of destiny and the daughter of Enki, the god of wisdom. She brought many gifts from her father to her people on Earth. Some of her gifts are making wise decisions, soothing desolate hearts, writing, and the ability to be alluring. Because she is a moon goddess, she is magnetic.

She is the Queen of Heaven, who had to make the descent into the underworld, like Persephone. One by one, she passed through seven gates, removing a piece of clothing as she went until she faced the underworld and was turned into a corpse. There she lay for three days and nights until she was sprinkled with the food of life and the water of life. In order to make her ascent back to her heavens, she had to provide a replacement for herself.

Another one of Inanna's tasks is to outwit her father, Enki, the god of wisdom, and get him to give her the sacred *Me's*. This is no easy task and yet Inanna is able to do it. She is also able to save her lover Dumuzi from a lifetime in the underworld due to her great love for him. Inanna's story of her love for Dumuzi is one of the first recorded love stories in the world. It is two thousand years older than the Bible.

Inanna is of medium height—sometimes on the short side—and would be considered overweight by today's impossibly thin standards! She has large, pendulous breasts, a large belly, wide hips, and big thighs. She has long, dark hair and almond-shaped black eyes.

Inanna's Story

How she got the Me's from her father for humankind

Enki, the god of wisdom, called his servant to him.

"Quick, make me the best butter cake you can prepare—one using our finest ingredients—and bring me some water and beer, for my beloved daughter Inanna is coming to visit and we must prepare a feast in her honor."

Inanna arrived at Eridu, the holy city of her father, wearing a beautiful crown of gold inlaid with diamond stars upon her long, ebony hair.

"I have come to Eridu to honor the god of wisdom," she announced. Enki's servant led her through the great hall to the holy table and bid her to sit down.

"Here, my lady, we have set the table for you, for we were awaiting your arrival. Eat this fine butter cake and drink this beer and water laid out especially for you."

Enki entered the room and eyed his daughter, marveling at her beauty. "Inanna, my beloved, how well you look. Please drink some more beer and we shall drink to your good health."

So the servant refilled their goblets and they drank together in silence. Before each bronze cup was emptied, the servant refilled it with more beer. Cup after cup they consumed, until Enki was quite intoxicated.

Enki lifted his goblet toward his daughter and intoned, "A blessing to you, dear daughter. I shall give you three gifts. The first, I give you the blessing of high priestess. The second, I bestow upon you the right of godship; the third, I crown you with kingship itself."

Inanna gravely raised her cup and eyed her father with a measuring look. She drank lustily and replied, "I accept."

They drank some more again in silence and presently Enki offered a second toast:

"A blessing to you, dear daughter, I shall give you three more gifts. The first I give you is the gift of truth, the second I give you is the ability to descend and ascend to the underworld, and the third I give you is the gift of wondrous love-making!"

Again Inanna raised her cup to her father and said, "I accept."

They drank even more beer and by this time Enki was drunk and feeling even more generous. He offered a third toast.

"A blessing to you, dear daughter. I give you joy and sorrow and the gift of wise judgment. Many are the roads you will take, many are the decisions you must make."

Inanna raised her cup in thanks.

"I accept," she said.

They continued to drink and Enki continued to give Inanna his blessings. She accepted each and every one of them with much gratitude, knowing that it was Enki's intoxication that caused him to be so generous. She was careful not to drink as much as he and her head was still fairly clear, with her wits about her.

By the end of the evening, Enki had bestowed upon her many more gifts from the divine realm. He gave her the gifts of music, of waging war and plundering cities, of heroism and power, of creating strife and soothing words that could calm strife. And he gave her the ability to bless families with children.

Finally, Enki called to his servant. "See my daughter out. Make sure she and all the gifts I have given her from the *Me's* safely reach the city of Uruk, where she lives."

"Yes, my lord," said the servant, and with that he escorted Inanna to the dock where her vessel, the Boat of Heaven, was anchored.

He helped her to load her precious cargo into the boat and watched carefully as the boat left the dock, setting sail for Uruk, the holy city of Inanna. In the meantime, Enki took himself off to bed and slept soundly throughout the night.

The next morning Enki arose with a pounding headache, his stomach sick and his mouth dry. His head was groggy with beer for most of the day. By evening he was feeling well enough to arise from his bed. He got up and immediately went to look for his great treasures, all the sacred gifts that were his as god of wisdom. However, they were nowhere to be seen.

The king searched high and low, throughout his castle and then through the holy city of Eridu, but to no avail. The divine gifts were gone. Finally he returned to his castle in a foul temper.

"Servant," he bellowed. "Come here at once!"

His servant came to him.

"Where are my precious things? Where are my treasures? My priesthood, my godship, my kingship, heroism, power. . . . Where have they all gone?"

"Why, my lord," the servant answered, shocked. "You gave them all to your daughter, Inanna, last night. Do you not remember?"

Enki glared at his servant. "Where the hell is Inanna now?" he demanded.

"Why, she has sailed to Uruk on the Boat of Heaven," exclaimed the servant. "You asked me to ensure she returned home safely!"

"Bring her back!" roared Enki. "Bring her back at once! Right this minute! Bring her back and all those damn gifts with her!"

"But sir," the servant implored. "She nears her own city, how can I stop her?"

Enki fussed and fumed and thought for several moments. Finally he called to him the Enkun, hairy creatures that could fly through the air.

"Take my servant to my dratted daughter Inanna who is right now sailing on her Boat of Heaven along with all *my* gifts!" he commanded. "Bring them back to me immediately!"

The Enkun lifted Enki's servant up under their hairy arms, and flew without a moment's delay to the Boat of Heaven.

From the deck, Inanna stood looking toward her city. There were only a few feet to go until her boat would be docked. On the quay she saw her faithful servant Ninshubar, the warrior woman, waiting for her. Behind Ninshubar were a number of her faithful subjects.

The Enkun surrounded Inanna's boat and dropped Enki's servant on deck.

"Your father most urgently commands that you return with his precious gifts to Eridu," cried the servant. "He wishes his gifts to be restored to him, and his order must be obeyed."

However Inanna had no intention of delivering the gifts back to her father.

"He breaks faith with me," she swore. "My father *gave* me the precious gifts. I did not steal them like some thief in the night. He bestowed them upon me. He has broken his honor and he has lied! I will not return them!"

Suddenly, the Enkun seized the Boat of Heaven and lifted it effortlessly into their arms to begin the long journey back to Eridu.

"Help me, Ninshubar!" screamed Inanna. "Fight with me, my faithful warrior!"

Together Inanna and Ninshubar let out howling battle cries and summoned up the powers of the wind. With their hands they directed the wind toward the Enkun. The force of the wind sent the Enkun reeling through the air. They dropped the boat back into the water, and the deadly wind sent the Enkun all the way back to Eridu.

But, the god of wisdom would not give up so easily. He commanded his giants to reach down and capture the Boat of Heaven. Enki then ordered his sea monster to seize the boat from below. But Ninshubar wrested it free from the monster's jaws and Inanna pushed the giants over so they toppled into the sea, splashing and fussing among themselves.

Ninshubar and Inanna fought fiercely to overcome each attempt Enki made to take back the things he had given his daughter.

At last, battle-worn and weary, Ninshubar and Inanna sailed the Boat of Heaven through the gates of the sacred city of Uruk.

"Let there be great joy and celebration in the city," cried Inanna, "for I bring with me the gifts of my father, Enki, god of wisdom!"

Back in Eridu, Enki awaited his servant's return. "Where are my precious gifts now?" he asked.

"The lady Inanna has already delivered them to the sacred temple of Uruk," answerd the servant. "At this moment she is presenting them to the people of Uruk."

"My daughter has fought courageously," noted Enki. "I have raised her well. Let her keep what I gave her.

"After all," he mused, "as allies we are stronger than as enemies." Plus Enki knew his drunkenness was partially to blame for his generosity. Perhaps it was time, after all, for him to pass on his mantle of power if he could not uphold it responsibly.

Inanna happily showed the people of Uruk all the wonderful gifts that the god of wisdom had bestowed upon her. In celebration, the people danced and sang in the streets.

When Enki, the god of wisdom, heard of the celebration, he pronounced another blessing, this time to all the people of Uruk, including Inanna, for she had shown that she was truly worthy of receiving his gifts. So Enki gave a prayer that they be blessed with prosperity and joy.

And so it was that Inanna came to share the divine gifts from her father with the mortals she so loved.

The Gift of Divine Wisdom

One of the gifts Enki gave Inanna was the gift of wisdom. To tune into divine wisdom there are many tools you can use. Divination tools, such as tarot cards, pendulums, and rune stones, are all accessories you can use to tune into your divine wisdom.

You can use divine wisdom for all sorts of things, from making an important decision to facing the unknown when you feel like all your resources have been taken from you to receiving goddess guidance about your future.

My favorite divination tool is the tarot. I have many different decks. To use the tarot, you need to buy a deck of tarot cards. There are many kinds of decks on the market. Choose one that has pictures you like. There are angel cards, animal cards, goddess cards (my favorite!), rune cards, traditional tarot, fairy cards, and even crystal and flower cards. Check them out in the New Age section of a bookstore.

How to Learn the Tarot

Once you have your cards, get a notepad and take the cards out one at a time. Look at the first card; what do you see in the card? What does it look like is happening in the card? What story is it telling you? What kind of emotions does it conjure up? Write your answers down in your notepad. Go through the entire pack, a few cards at each sitting, writing down the answers for each card.

Think of each card as a window into the spirit world. Sometimes it will seem as if the picture in the card is moving—like watching a mini movie. Think of a question you would like to know the answer to. Don't ask yes or no questions, ask questions like "What would be the outcome of doing . . ." or "Show me what I need to do about . . ."

When you have a question in mind, shuffle the cards and say a prayer to Inanna, like "Dear Goddess, please give me the perfect card that gives me the best answer to the question I seek." Then pull a card from the deck. Sometimes you may feel warmth or buzzing around a certain card, or sometimes one card may "accidentally" drop out.

Read what that card says. Look at the picture and read what it is saying to you, using the questions above as a guideline. You can use the instructions in the tarot guide that comes with the cards, too. However, I find it best to go on your own intuition. Sometimes the same card can change meaning, depending on the situation. You will know each time you read it what it is saying to you at that particular moment.

Finding Your Life Purpose

Inanna is a goddess who weighs your life to see the measure of it at the end of your lifetime. She is the goddess to go to for help in remembering your divine life purpose—the reason why you chose to incarnate at this time.

You have three different life purposes:

1. Your Planetary Life Purpose

This is the way you are supposed to share your talents with the world—the legacy you will leave behind, the meaningful work you will do that makes a difference in the world. Some examples of this are being a writer, an environmentalist, a teacher, or a public speaker. Your career may be one way you express your planetary work. Hobbies or charity work are other ways. Even just being a good person and extending kindness to others on a daily basis is a valid way of living out your divine planetary purpose.

To discover your planetary purpose, pray:

Dear Goddess

Help me to remember the reason I chose to incarnate at this time

Remind me of the gifts I have to share with the world

2. Your Personal Life Purpose

These are the personal life lessons you came here to learn. All of us have weak spots, areas in our personality that we would like to strengthen. You can tell what your personal life purpose is by seeing what kinds of situations keep popping up in your life. Perhaps you find yourself often doing things you don't want to do or giving others too much of yourself. If this is the case, your personal life purpose may be to learn how to set boundaries.

Maybe you find yourself being rejected over and over. In this case, your personal life purpose may be to learn self-love and self-acceptance so you can believe you are worthy of acceptance, and seek out people who will mirror this back to you.

Perhaps you are incredibly hard on yourself and often beat yourself up, torturing yourself unmercifully in your mind. Your personal life purpose may be to learn to be kind to yourself.

Your personal life purpose includes the type of life you seek to live. Having children or not having children is all part of your personal life purpose. Being married or choosing to remain single or having multiple relationships over your lifetime may be part of your personal life purpose.

I knew at a very early age that part of my personal life purpose was to have children and to be married. I dreamed about those things constantly. Six years before my first son was born, I knew what he would look like and what his name would be. Marriage was also extremely important to me. I love being married—even though my dreams of what marriage would be like were a little off-balance due to all the romance novels I read! However, despite all the trials and tribulations I have faced within my marriage, I still love being married.

Coping with a handicap or chronic illness also falls into the category of personal life purpose. Learning to live with any kind of disability or setback causes you to grow as a person. Obstacles are challenges that stretch you to reach new heights. They are gifts, although they may not seem like it at the time. However, it is what you do with your challenges that are important. You have the choice to let them limit you or to learn from them and use your new knowledge to make your life even more wonderful.

I know a girl who has diabetes. When she was first diagnosed, she was very scared and angry. As time went on, she discovered all kinds of things about her body and how to take good care of it that she would never have known if she hadn't been diabetic. Stories abound of people who have been seriously injured who have done amazing things with their lives.

Goddess Workout

What do you think your personal life purpose might be at this time?

What situations seem to keep cropping up in your life?

How could they be lessons from which you can learn something?

What actions do you need to take to change the situations?

What do you dream about doing when you become an adult? What pictures come to mind? What would you like to be doing in ten years' time, for example?

3. *Your Divine Life Purpose*

These are the lessons your spirit is here to learn. Growing spiritually is a part of your divine life purpose. Learning compassion or forgiveness, empathy or understanding are all lessons that stretch our spirits. Learning divine love and how to love are important lessons, too.

Sometimes events happen that seem absolutely horrible or senseless. Injustice occurs and situations happen that may seem like no good can possibly come from them. For example, there was nothing good about the World Trade Center being destroyed. Other injustices that occur, like rape, sexual abuse, infidelity, theft, injuries, bullying, violence, or betrayal, are the same—there is nothing good about them. The events themselves will never be "right" or "just" but, once again, it is what you do afterwards that is important. The outcome can be larger than the event.

Those types of events are life changing. However, again you have a choice. You can let them destroy you or you can use them to make you stronger. You can let them define you or you can decide you are going to define your life by your own standards.

Nothing can destroy your spirit, even though it may feel like it is broken or has disappeared at times. But your spirit is stronger than any situation and will live long after the body is dead.

Good things can happen that cause you to grow spiritually, too, like when someone does something incredibly kind and you are touched by his or her generosity. Or when you meet someone who becomes a mentor or role model for you. This may cause you to try things you never would have thought you could accomplish previously.

Other important divine life purposes include learning how to manifest good things in your life, learning how to banish bad things, and learning how to use your spiritual power.

What are some of the things you have learned spiritually recently?

If you are unsure of your divine life purpose, simply light a candle and pray to Inanna:

Dear Goddess

I seem to have forgotten my life purpose

Please help me to remember why I am here

Awaken my spirit to remember its true purpose

Let me hear the whisperings of my spirit

When bad things happen, help me to view the situation with my spiritual sight

When good things happen, remind me to give gratitude

Let me know that you are always with me

Guiding me, loving me, and helping me

By the way, in case you are wondering, it is not God or the Goddess who cause bad things to happen. People sometimes ask why bad things happen. Well, we all have free will and sometimes people choose, for whatever reason, to do bad stuff. Sometimes you may just happen to be on the receiving end of bad stuff happening. I do not believe that this is all part of the Goddess's divine plan for your life that you be made to suffer. But I do believe that it is part of the Goddess's plan for you to help you get through it. There is no value in staying stuck in suffering.

Your Divine Gifts

We are all given divine gifts that we bring into the world with us. It is our Goddess-given duty to utilize these skills to the best of our ability. Many times people feel unworthy of developing their talents or following their dreams. However, the Goddess wants you to use your gifts and share your talents with the world. Not using them serves no one—least of all you! Sometimes people let fear of not being good enough stand in their way. Fears of not having the resources, the time, the know-how, or the money can be a block to pursuing your dreams.

Sometimes fear of not being worthy to receive can be a block, too, like you are afraid to charge people for your services, or you downplay any compliments you receive for a job well done. If this is the case, think of yourself as giving to the world when you share your gifts, and in return be willing for the world to give back to you in terms of money or acknowledgment or whatever it is you need or desire.

Your dreams are gifts from the Goddess, and the Goddess fully supports you in your undertaking to make your dreams come true. All she asks is that you ask for help and listen for guidance and take action every day toward making your dreams come true. She will help you with everything you need. And when one door closes, she will always open another.

....

Goddess Workout

What are your divine gifts? What are the things you most love to do? Perhaps you have a special gift of empathy and are good at helping other people sort out their problems. Perhaps you love music and would love to play professionally. Maybe you are good at writing or have a desire to write books or magazine articles. You may love sports and wish to be a successful athlete.

To discover your divine gifts, answer the following questions:

1. What do you love to do?

2. What do you seem to have a natural aptitude for?

3. What secret dreams and desires do you have?

4. If you could be anything, what would that be?

5. What do other people compliment you about?

When you feel unworthy or insecure about your abilities, say a prayer to Inanna:

Dearest Goddess

I ask that you give me courage to follow my dreams

Please help me to use my divine gifts for their highest good

Lead me to the people, places, and resources that will enhance my talents

Show me the actions I need to take to utilize my gifts

Give me the courage to take these actions

And remove any blocks or fears that hold me back

Thank you, Dear Goddess

And so it is

Amen

Inanna's Glamour

- Smokey eyes

- Midnight-blue clothes

- Silver glitter

- Her makeup is dramatic and magnetic (she is very alluring)

- Makeup gel that has glow-in-the-dark stars and moons inside it

Makeup

Inanna's skin is a coppery color, so use a foundation that gives your skin a bronze glow. If you have dark skin, so much the better for this glamour. If you have pale skin, try a bronzer gently shimmered over your face.

Line your eyes with dark blue or black eyeliner. Take the eyeliner all the way from the inner corner of the eye to the outer corner of the eye and extend it upward toward your brow bone. Apply a smoky gray shadow to your eyelids and a silver shadow to your brow bone. Define your eyebrows with black or dark brown eye pencil, depending on your coloring. Make them look bold. The eyeliner and the brows are the most striking aspect of Inanna's makeup look.

Line your lips with a fuchsia or magenta lip pencil, and fill them in with lip gloss of the same color.

Use a pale pink blush on the apples of your cheeks, and apply a touch of highlighter to the upper part of your cheekbone.

Clothing

Try a long blue dress with silver jewelry. Dark denim jeans are good, too.

If you have a beautiful necklace or choker, wear that, as Inanna wore beautiful necklaces to show that she was a queen.

Ceremony

This ceremony is for trusting your intuition and using discernment, the wisdom of Inanna.

Get dressed in your goddess costume and makeup for Inanna.

Put your jewelry on, and any woodsy fragrance you may have, like sandalwood. Put some relaxing music on the stereo.

Stand in the middle of your room. Close your eyes and visualize a circle of silver stars about two feet away from you, all around you, at tummy level. Hold your arms up toward the sky in a *V* shape. Stand with your feet firmly placed on the ground about two feet apart.

Breathe deeply through your nose to a count of four and hold for four seconds, then breathe out through your mouth to a count of four. Do this four-by-four breath five times.

See an imaginary opening in the top of your crown. Imagine a silver liquid elixir of wisdom pouring into this opening. Inanna is standing in front of you, holding a beautiful jug filled with this magical elixir, which she pours into your crown.

Pray:

Inanna, goddess of wisdom

Fill me with your divine inspiration

Help me see clearly

The situation at hand

Guide me with your divine knowledge

Dear Goddess

As you say the prayer, you may feel a tingling in your third-eye area so you know that Inanna is activating your crown chakra and your brow chakra so that you will be a clear and open channel for divine wisdom.

Feel her power and wisdom building within you now. Bring your palms together with your arms still stretched above your head, and inhale as you do. Then extend your arms outwards into the *V* again, exhaling. Repeat this movement over and over while you imagine the wisdom of Inanna flowing into you. Keep it up for three minutes. This will increase the flow of *prana* (spiritual energy) into your body and will stimulate your heart and glandular system.

Then get out your goddess journal. Write a question to Inanna about something that has been troubling you or a decision that you need to make. Ask her what to do, listen to what she says, and then write down her answer. Don't worry if you feel like you are making it up. Just write it down anyway. Write down, too, what your gut says about the situation. What is your gut feeling? What is your intuition trying to tell you?

Inanna's Tasks for You

- Get a tarot deck and practice using it. Follow the suggestions given in this chapter.

- Spend one day as Inanna—how does it feel to be a goddess of wisdom? Write about your experience in your goddess journal.

◆ Practice discernment. Do this by choosing a situation that has been troubling you and asking Inanna to help you take a step backwards so you can view it from a different perspective. Imagine you are flying above your life, getting a bird's-eye view of the whole situation.

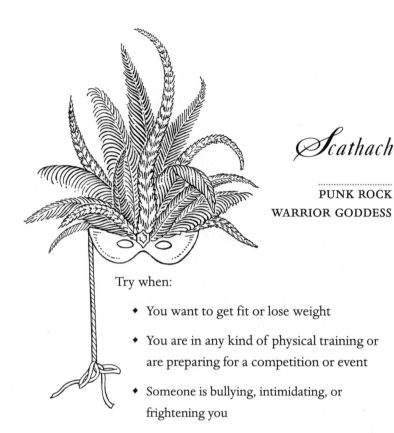

Scathach

PUNK ROCK
WARRIOR GODDESS

Try when:

- ◆ You want to get fit or lose weight

- ◆ You are in any kind of physical training or
  are preparing for a competition or event

- ◆ Someone is bullying, intimidating, or
  frightening you

Scathach (pronounced *skath-ark*) is the original punk rocker.
She is a Celtic warrior with her own army. She is tall, with
bright orange hair that sticks up in spikes all over her head.
Her clothing is plaid and she takes much pleasure in dressing
herself brightly for battle. Scathach kicks butt. She isn't afraid
of anybody or anything. She doesn't look kindly upon sissies.

Getting to her house is an ordeal all of its own. That way
she can ensure only people worthy of her time get to see her.
Her body is as battered as her weapons, bearing scars from
head to toe, each one telling a story, a badge of pride from another battle successfully won. Tattoos adorn her hard, muscular body.

Scathach has a camp where she trains young girls and
boys to be great warriors just like her. Her encampment is the
original boot camp. This lady is tough. If you want to train

with her, you have to be prepared to die for her. All her students are fighters in her army, which meant if someone had a bone to pick with Scathach, they had a bone to pick with you.

Scathach's Story

How she trained Cuchulain

Scathach was the most famous warrior in the entire land. People came from as far away as France to her training camp on the Isle of Skye in Scotland for the chance to train with her. Those she trained became ferocious warriors and were greatly feared by others.

On this particular day, Scathach stood at her watching post and observed the young man approaching her isle. She knew he was coming because she was a goddess and she had been waiting for him.

This was the master apprentice named Cuchulain that she must train. Word of his glory and battle rage had spread throughout the land.

She watched his approach with keen interest to see how he would manage the perilous bridge he must cross to get to her isle. She had made her fortress nearly impenetrable so only those worthy of her training would succeed in crossing.

Cuchulain goes to cross the bridge. It is a dark, stormy day. As he steps onto the bridge, it sways violently, almost throwing him off into the swirling vortex of sea below. Shocked, he falls back onto solid ground. The wind whips painfully across his face.

Scathach watches him with a smile upon her lips. "Oh yes, cocky one, it is not so easy as you first thought."

Cuchulain frowns. He hasn't come all this way to be put out by some dumb bridge. Plus the whole reason he is here is because of a promise made to his true love's dad. If he trains with Scathach, he will be allowed to marry his lovely Emer.

He takes a deep breath and, with a picture of Emer vividly in his mind, faces the bridge.

He hears the snickers of those already on the stronghold. More than anything, he *hates* being laughed at. He closes his eyes; a familiar, warm sensation begins to burn in his belly. Rage ignites within him. Let them laugh. He lets the rage fuel his body, moving from his belly outwards. He loses his sense of time and focuses only on the task at hand—getting his body across the bridge onto the island.

Scathach is curious. She had heard of this young one's battle rage, the mad frenzy that comes upon him when he is in a fight. She watches as he takes five slow steps backwards, like a cat backing up from its prey before the attack. She sees him breathe slowly and deeply, his eyes squinting with determination, glazing over as if drugged. "He is in another world," she thinks to herself. "Yes, this one has power, but does he know how to use it wisely? Only time will tell of that."

In an instant he is running, and with one giant leap he lands with one foot on the middle of the bridge, then springboards himself upwards into another leap like a fish out of water. His body propels forward with the grace of a spear thrusting toward its target and then he lands perfectly, two feet ajar, right in front of Scathach.

The warrior steps back, not allowing her bemusement to show. *Never let your mask slip* is the first training of a warrior. *Act, don't react.* "I see you made it, little one," she says dryly. "Is this your usual way of appearing?"

Cuchulain is mortified at his rudeness. He hadn't thought to approach the fortress by knocking on the door. Well, leaping over her stronghold had kind of prevented that from happening anyway. But it was of tantamount importance that she be willing to train him. If not, he would have to forget about marrying Emer, and he wasn't about to let *that* happen.

He let himself take in the woman before him before deciding how best to make amends. Scathach noticed his poise and inwardly commended him. A good warrior must take the measure of what is before him.

She was all muscle, he noticed. Lean, firm, and lithe. She was smaller than he had imagined, more feminine. Somehow he had thought he would see a woman in a man's body. But not this woman—for all her muscles and prowess, there was no forgetting she was a woman. Her muscles curved in all the right places and she was strong, of that there was no doubt. Her body was as taut as a rope tied between two chariots, each pulling in the opposite direction.

The thought flickered through his mind of what it would be like to hold a woman like that, one so compact yet sensual, contained but wild. Scathach noticed the flicker of lust sweep across his face. She smiled inwardly. Part of her job as teacher required her to train him in the arts of love as well as the arts of battle, for love and battle go hand in hand, as does life and death. The first would be pure pleasure. But she was a hard taskmaster. He would have to earn his skills. "So," she thought. "Let the training begin."

And tough training it was. For months and months Scathach drove Cuchulain mercilessly. Every day he learned new battle skills. She taught him thirty ways to land on his feet, avoiding his enemies' sword thrusts. Thirty ways to pierce his enemies' skin with his sword she also taught, and how to dance on the rim of a spinning shield while throwing a spear. She made him run faster, jump higher, think quicker, and be better than he had ever been before. And she taught him how to face his opponents. "More people are defeated with intimidation than with weapons," she instilled.

Now Scathach had a mighty weapon named the Gae Bulga, which was an invincible spear. Although she had owned it for a long time, she had never been able to use it. The spear had strange and magical powers. It chose to whom it would belong.

One morning Scathach took Cuchulain out to train and handed him the Gae Bulga, watching to see what would happen. As Cuchulain gripped the spear in his hand, he felt a jolt of power surge through his body. The spear was alive. It knew him. Cuchulain listened carefully. He could hear the spear telling him exactly how it wanted to be thrown.

Scathach watched carefully. "You hold in your hands a powerful weapon, Cuchulain. It never misses its mark. No mortal has ever been able to use it until now. It has claimed you. Use it wisely."

For years, Scathach had been at war with her sister Ayfa, whom she had once trained. "We must put this battle to end, once and for all," said the great teacher. "You must fight her, Cuchulain, and put your new skills to the test."

On the morning of the battle, Ayfa looked over the young warrior who had been presented to fight her. "Surely you jest, sister," she scoffed. "I will make mincemeat of this babe in five easy strokes!"

Cuchulain's face darkened. "I shall fight your entire army single-handedly, woman," he boasted. "Then we'll see who is making mincemeat out of whom!"

Ayfa pulled out her dagger. The fight began. In five steps Cuchulain had knocked her unconscious. He would not kill a woman. One by one he took on the rest of her warriors, and one by one they fell. At the end of the day the field was a bloody mess.

Satisfied, Scathach took her pupil home to a hero's feast. She had taught him well.

Women Warriors in Celtic Society

Celtic women were renowned for their strength and ferociousness. They were not just stay-at-home women who kept themselves busy with darning and cooking and let the men take care of warring.

There were lots of women warriors in Celtic history and mythology. There was Queen Boadicea, whom we will meet in a later chapter. She led a revolt against the Romans when they raped her daughters and publicly flogged her. There was Grania Ni Mhaille, a famous Irish pirate (one of my favorite heroines) who lived at the same time as Queen Elizabeth I. Grania protected her lands from invaders and led a ship with a crew of pirates (read more about Grania in Morgan Llywelyn's wonderful historical novel *Grania: She-King of the Irish Seas* [Ivy Books, 1987]). There was the powerful warrior queen Maeve, who led a battle against Cuchulain in the famous Irish tale of the cattle raid of Cooley. And there was the Morrigan, goddess of war and fertility, who appeared as a crow on the battlefield, signaling death and rebirth.

To be a warrior in Celtic society was a great honor. Warriors were part of the "white collar" class of professionals and garnered utmost respect. Warriors trained for many years and took great pride in their strength and skills. Both men and women could train as warriors, and children could be sent to train at an early age with a skilled warrior.

Women were required by law to defend their property if necessary. Sometimes they went to war themselves or led their armies into battle. Sometimes they employed armies to battle for them.

Roman writers often commented on Celtic women's strength. Siculus said that Celtic women were not only equal to their husbands in height and build, but rivaled them in strength as well. Marcelinus said that Celtic women were stronger than their husbands by far! He stated that a whole band of foreigners would be unable to cope if fighting against a Celtic man whose wife was fighting with him!

Warfare and learning battle skills were a high priority in daily Celtic life. When Cuchulain went to train with Scathach, he learned many skills, like thirty different foot movements to avoid being hit by an enemy's sword, and thirty different ways to cut open an enemy's body with his sword. In Celtic society there was a big emphasis on learning battle skills, strategies, and fighting techniques and weapons. Elaborate codes of honor were in place to ensure fair play. Spiritual practices were an important part of fighting—the Celts believed a god or goddess could come and aid them when they fought. They often called upon the help of a particular goddess before battle. They also believed their weapons could be inhabited by gods and goddesses and could have magical properties, like Cuchulain's famous spear the Gae Bulga, which never missed a target, and King Arthur's sword Excalibur.

Your Personal Warrior Training

Call on Scathach for any kind of physical training. If you want to get fit or you are an athlete and have an important event coming up, get Scathach to help you. She is the goddess of competition. Even if you are not particularly athletic but have a sports event to participate in, call on Scathach. She will help you even if you absolutely dread any kind of physical exertion.

Training the Body

An adept warrior must be physically and mentally fit. In Celtic society it was illegal for a man to be overweight, and he would be fined accordingly—kind of like getting a traffic ticket. This may seem harsh to us today, but remember that Celtic society was a warrior society. The survival of the tribe depended on the fitness of their warriors. Being a warrior was an honor that had to be continually worked at in order to keep the title, just like having a black belt in karate.

How much physical fitness have you been getting lately?

If you are involved in sports at school, you probably get quite a lot. If not, you may need to make an extra effort to get your body moving. I never did any exercises when I was in high school—I thought I was uncoordinated and so I hated sports. Looking back, I see I just didn't know how to move my body or breathe properly when exercising.

Having a good teacher can make all the difference to your exercise experience. If you have been shamed by others, don't let that put you off. See if you can find a kind teacher to get you started, or get a book or video out of the library in a sport you think you might enjoy and study some basic techniques. Keep it simple. You don't need to tell anyone what you are doing. Choose something that seems fun and easy—like power walking or dancing.

125

Exercise has many benefits. Regular exercise strengthens the body, giving you shapely muscles and overall endurance. It increases your stamina, your heart and lung capacity, and oxygenates the blood so you have more energy. Exercise speeds up your metabolism so you burn fat more efficiently. It stimulates your lymphatic system so toxins are eliminated from your body. Exercise has many emotional rewards as well as physical ones. During exercise, your body secretes natural antidepressants so you start to feel better if you have been feeling down. Getting twenty minutes of vigorous activity daily will clear your head and help you keep your emotions stable.

The benefits of regular exercise are:

- Increased self-esteem and confidence

- Extra energy

- Improved health

- Banished depression

- Emotional well-being

- Strength, endurance, and stamina

- Toned muscles

- Better coordination

Useful Exercise Tips

FIND AN EXERCISE YOU ENJOY

Swimming every day is silly if you hate water. So is joining a gym if you feel self-conscious about exercising in front of others. There are many different types of exercise, so choose one you like. Exercise can be as simple as going for a walk every morning, dancing to your favorite music on the stereo, or following a video on TV. Exercise does not have to be expensive or complicated to be effective.

SET REALISTIC GOALS

If you haven't exercised for a while, it is better to walk for twenty minutes each day instead of trying to jog for forty-five. If your goals are too hard for you to reach, you will be more likely to give up after a few days. Set small goals and make them more challenging as you become fitter.

EXERCISE EVERY DAY

Sticking to something is easier when it is part of your daily routine. Find a time that suits your schedule and stick to it. First thing in the morning works well for me. Some of my friends like to work out after school or in the evening.

USE VISUALIZATION WHILE EXERCISING

Imagine you are a warrior woman training with Scathach. Imagine you have to fight fierce opponents or lead your tribe into battle. Imagine your body becoming fit and powerful as you move. Imagine your heart opening and your mind expanding as you stretch.

Try an exercise that uses all your power. Try slamming a racquetball against a wall for twenty minutes. Try going for a run and imagining Scathach is pushing you further forward. You are a warrior woman in training. Every day you must work your body to increase your strength and power.

Training the Mind

Your mind is your most valuable asset as a warrior. Scathach told Cuchulain that more people were defeated by intimidation than by weapons. What she meant is that mental battle tactics are more important than physical ones. You must train your mind and emotions every day to stay in peak condition. Mental and emotional fitness is just as important as physical fitness.

Boasting

Boasting was an art form in Celtic society. Before going into battle, warriors would describe in excruciating detail exactly what they planned to do to their enemies. This technique was to induce fear and self-doubt in their opponents. The Celts knew if they gained a mental advantage over their foes, they would be easier to defeat physically. I saw this illustrated recently when watching the Olympics. A coach was talking about his Russian gymnast, whom he described as a "10" in physical ability but as being less than a "10" in mental ability. Sometimes at the most crucial moment of the gymnast's performance, he would have a flicker of self-doubt. Invariably this self-doubt would lead to him making a mistake. Even though his body could perform the routine perfectly, his mind would trip him up.

Practice Focus and Determination

Bring your goal into focus. If you want to win a competition, see yourself winning. If someone is intimidating you, start seeing yourself intimidating him or her in your imagination. Make mental pictures of yourself as strong, powerful, and competent. See yourself as succeeding. Hold on to this picture. Don't let yourself think about failing, no matter how badly things seem to be going. Always picture success.

Don't build up obstacles. If a worry thought comes to mind, simply choose to focus on a success thought. Whenever self-doubt arises, deliberately voice a positive thought to cancel it. Last week I had to give a speech at a bookstore. I was so scared, I thought I was going to be sick. That day I decided to "practice what I preach." Each time a fear thought rose in my mind, I would say out loud: "We're not doing fear today." And you know what? It worked.

Imagine Scathach is actually with you, helping you. See her as your constant companion, helping you and standing up with you. Remind yourself throughout the day that the Goddess is with you and nothing can defeat you. Say, "I believe in a power far greater than myself. The power of the Goddess flows through me. I can do all things through the power of the Goddess." See her strengthening you and see her power flowing through you. Make your body and mind a conduit for goddess power.

Have faith in the Goddess!

128

I often use the pronoun "we" instead of "I" if I have a scary situation in front of me. I do this to remind myself I am not alone—that I have the power of the Goddess, my ancestors, my guardian angels, and the spirit world right along with me.

How to Cope with Bullies

Bullying is unfortunately a situation that affects many teenagers these days. I talked with my friend David Brown, Deputy Sheriff First Class and martial arts Sifu, who has had a lot of experience dealing with bullies during his thirty-one years on the police force, and this is what he said.

People need to understand the mindset of a bully before they can bully-proof their children. Typically a bully is the youngest in the family, with older siblings and self-esteem issues. Often you cannot pacify these kids, as they tend to have no conscience about what they do or who they harm. Usually they are acting out in anger something that has happened to them in their immediate life. Trying to reason with their parents can be difficult, too, as the parents are often in denial about their kid's behavior and may minimize it by saying, "Well, you must have done something to provoke him or her" or "My child would never do anything like that."

Unfortunately, many teenage bullies are in the early stages of exhibiting anti-social personality disorder. So when you are dealing with a bully most likely you are not dealing with someone whom you can reason with like a regular person. They tend to have no concept of the consequences of their behavior and a lack of conscience so when they have their mind set on hurting someone, they will do it regardless of the cost.

However, that said, if you are in a situation where someone is intimidating you or threatening you in any way, there are many steps you can take to ensure your safety. You have the right to be safe wherever you are, and there are laws in place to protect you.

If someone is bullying you this is what you need to do:

Tell an Adult that You Trust

You must tell a parent or a schoolteacher. As soon as someone verbally threatens you, tell your parents. Don't feel silly for feeling intimidated by someone, or feel like you can deal with it on your own. The sooner you let an adult know, then they can take action to ensure your safety. If the bully is threatening you at school or on the school bus, your parents or a trusted adult can report it to the school. If any violence does occur at a later date, then in most jurisdictions the school is liable, so by making them aware of the situation they can take action to protect you. If the bullying is taking place outside of school, then your parents must file a police report. If the police are reluctant to take a report, ask to talk to the supervisor and tell the supervisor you want a report filed. Make sure you take the name of the policeman who filed the report, and the date. Also take the name of the teacher whom you reported the bullying to and the date. David says you must start a paper trail immediately.

Ask the Bully Why They Are Being Mean to You

Sometimes you can reason with a bully and find out why they have it in for you. Even if you do come to some kind of understanding, you must still tell an adult what has happened. If the bully says they want you to give them lunch money for protection, or any of your belongings—videos, clothing, Gameboys, or whatever—this is extortion and it is illegal, so you must tell your parents and they must file a police report. Don't think that by giving the bully what they want, you will get them off your back. If a bully wants to hurt you, he or she will hurt you and will probably have no remorse about it.

Remember, This Is a Cycle of Violence

The bully cycle of violence is very similar to the domestic cycle of violence where husbands beat up their wives (or vice versa). Bullies may say things like, "If I beat you up it's because you deserve it, and if you tell anyone I'll just beat you up harder." Teens who are being threatened start to develop a certain mindset. They start to think "Well, I must have done something wrong to be in this situation." This is absolutely not true. You do not deserve to be on the receiving end of someone else's violence.

130

Teens begin to display certain symptoms when they are in an ongoing bullying situation. You may suffer from depression, stop being motivated, your schoolwork may suffer, you may stop taking care of yourself, and you may not want to go out of the house alone. That is why it is so important to tell someone as soon as you are threatened in any way.

Check the Laws In Your State

In many states, if anyone verbally threatens to harm you—whether they say "I'm going to beat the crap out of you" or intimidate you in anyway—this is illegal and it is a misdemeanor. If they repeatedly threaten you verbally, this is harassment, even if they never touch you. If they lay their hands on you in any way, whether by pushing you, poking you in the chest with their finger, hitting or touching you, this is assault, even if you are not physically hurt—it is still a criminal offense. If you are physically hurt, then this is aggravated battery and it is a very serious criminal offense.

Please take bullying seriously. The sooner you take action and get help from adults, the sooner you can prevent the situation from worsening. You do not have to handle this on your own. When I was a teen there was a girl who bullied me for a year. I spent that year in terror because I was too afraid to tell anyone. Finally I told my mother and she took action to stop the bullying. If I had talked about it sooner I could have saved myself a year of misery. Speak up—people can't help you unless they know what is going on.

Bullies exist in every culture, according to David. But you can take steps to prevent them from harming you. If someone is bullying you, intimidating you, or just plain frightening you, remember that Scathach is the "kick butt" goddess. She excels in single combat—one against one—and has even been known to take on whole armies. With Scathach on your side, you can throw your fear away.

Magical Tattooing

Scathach's body was adorned with tattoos. This was a common Celtic practice. Tattooing has long been used as a sacred spiritual practice in many cultures. In Asia, warrior men would tattoo their bodies and faces to protect themselves from large fish. Tattoos served as a protective shield and as a sacrifice to the supernatural. The design and position of the tattoo would vary according to the person's rank.

Tattoed mummies have been found in many parts of the world. One famous one is Amunet, who was a priestess of the goddess Hathor in ancient Egypt around 2000 B.C. Amunet had tattoos on her arms and thighs and above her belly button, which experts believe represented fertility and rejuvenation.

In New Zealand, Maori facial tattoos are called a *moko*. Both women and men tattooed their faces. When I was growing up in New Zealand, it was not common to see anyone with a moko because after the Pakeha (white people) came to New Zealand, this practice was almost abolished. Today many Maoris are choosing to continue the tradition of facial tattoos with traditional and modern designs.

Traditionally women tattooed their lips blue, which was considered a sign of beauty. They also tattooed their chins, and sometimes their cheeks and foreheads. The moko served as each person's unique signature. It described the rank of the person, their lineage, and their warrior status. When Maori chiefs had to sign land deed papers, they would draw their moko instead of writing their name.

Tattoos can serve many purposes. Warriors would use them for protection, like a magical shield engraved into their body. Tattoos can act as an amulet to draw something to you, like love, fertility, money, or creativity. They can also be a talisman to keep something from you—an enemy, worry, poor health, or bad luck.

They can tell a story of a transformation you have undergone or a rite of passage you have made. Or they can tell of your spiritual lineage or family heritage or your personal status. They can act as a goddess symbol, acknowledging that a particular goddess looks after you.

Getting a tattoo is a big decision and one you should wait until you are past your teenage years to make. Try experimenting with temporary tattoos instead. They are fun, cheap, and you can use different ones, depending on your need. Choose symbols that are meaningful to you, like maybe a rose or a heart if you want to attract love, or a Celtic design to invoke Scathach.

Scathach's Glamour

- Manic Panic temporary orange hair dye or orange Kool-Aid

- Vaseline or hair gel to make your hair stick up

- Temporary tattoos

- Some kind of plaid clothes—plaid pants, if possible, or a plaid scarf or skirt

- Sturdy shoes—Scathach is not the goddess to wear high heels. Doc Martens are perfect, as are Nikes or strong black or brown leather shoes

- Dark blue eyeliner (I like the kind with glitter in it)

- Lots of mascara

- A vest

- Cargo or army pants with a crop top

- A serious face—save your smiles for later

- A muscle T-shirt

- Chapstick for your lips

- A piece of jewelry that has a warrior feel to it—like a choker, a Celtic pendant, or an armband. The Celts loved neck torques and armbands. You can improvise with modern accessories, like sparkly chokers or armbands. Even a piece of gold jewelry is appropriate, as they loved gold, too.

- Power clothes—you can give Scathach a modern twist. Go for something modern, slick, and severe, like black tight pants and a black lycra long-sleeved shirt, or iron-gray pants and sweater. With this look you could wear black shoes with a clunky sole to make you appear taller—the taller, the better. Scathach likes to intimidate her enemies. But don't worry if you are naturally short—with Scathach you will seem taller.

133

This sacred ceremony involves trance dancing to raise the power of the Goddess. This is a great glamour to throw before you have to meet someone or something that intimidates you. Use it also before an important competition or when you are really mad—just dance your anger—or when you want to raise your own warrior energy. Try this if you have been battling depression—it's not called "battling" for nothing! When you bring out your personal power, it is hard to stay feeling depressed for very long.

Gather up the supplies you will need. Decide if you are going to dye your hair orange or not. Of course, Scathach's energy will still flow through you no matter what your hair color! I used to dye my hair with food coloring as it would just wash out the next day. Kool-Aid has the same effect. Manic Panic will last a bit longer, so you need to make more of a commitment to the color.

Now you are going to lay out your clothes and jewelry, then take a bath or shower. Once you are clean, wrap your hair in a towel and let's make-up.

Makeup

Before you apply any makeup, put some moisturizer on your face. Always apply moisturizer in upward strokes. Then apply sunscreen if it is daytime. Use sunscreen every day, even in winter. This will prevent you from getting wrinkles due to sun damage when you are older. I like to use Neutrogena sunblock lotion SPF 30.

Now it is time for foundation. You don't need foundation for this glamour, as Scathach's face has a healthy glow, so you could try tinted moisturizer as an alternative. Especially if you are going to be doing something athletic, you don't want foundation dripping down your face onto your clothes. But if you do want to wear foundation, choose a color in a shade close to your own skin color. Apply it with a damp sponge using gentle downward strokes. The reason for using downward strokes is because the fine hairs on your face grow downward and it looks weird if you apply foundation upwards.

Now we are going to apply brow pencil and eyeliner. Use a brow pencil in a color a shade darker than your eyebrows—you want your brows to look strong but not overly defined. Gently make little upward strokes with the pencil, following your natural eyebrow line, and blend, using your little finger. You can use a brown eye shadow as an alternative to a brow pencil. Dab a slanted brow brush into the shadow and brush over your brows.

Use eyeliner in a strong color like dark blue, forest green, black, or dark brown. You want your eyes to look fierce for this glamour. I like navy-blue eyeliner pencil with glitter in it—Bonne Bell makes a good one. Apply eyeliner, starting at the inner corner of your eyelid and extending it outward just past the corner of the outer eyelashes. Do the same underneath your eye. Make the line fairly wide and smudge it a bit with your little finger.

Then apply a dab of eyeliner in the crease between your eyelid and brow bone. Extend the liner from your outer lashes to the crease. Smudge this slightly too.

Now we are on to eye shadow. Celtic women wore eye shadow. They used berries to darken their eyes and to redden their lips. Choose an eye shadow in a berry color. If you want to go for a full-on punk rock look, use a red shadow or a hot pink one with flecks of gold, like L'Oreal's "Finch Kiss." But be prepared: this may make your eyes look really strange.

Okay, now apply blush, also in a berry color. For lips, go for a lipstick in a dramatic color like purple, wine, or blue. The Celts painted their bodies blue with woad before going into battle. And remember, Maori women tattooed their lips a bluish-green color.

Clothing

Scathach was the original punk rock chick, with her flaming orange hair and plaid pants.

If you don't want to go for the whole punk rock warrior look, you can tone it down. Omit the hair dye and choose jewelry and clothing that is applicable to you. This can include power dressing, like cargo pants with sneakers or workout gear. Ask Scathach for help—even goddesses like to experiment with different looks. See page 132's list for some ideas to get you started.

The main point to remember with Scathach is you need to be able to move your body easily. Scathach is a warrior and must be able to move her body quickly. So when you want to invoke her powers, you need to be able to move your body quickly, too.

Hairstyle

Celtic warriors used lime paste to make their hair stand up. Punk rockers use glue. I don't know about you, but I'm not too keen to try either one of those. You can use a maximum-hold gel to good effect. If you want to try making your hair stick straight up, like the ancient Celtic warriors, then you will need to use a strong adhesive. However, a messy, just-got-out-of-bed hairdo is perfectly adequate.

Scrunch-dry your hair by leaning over and tipping your head upside down. Scrunch handfuls of your hair as you dry it. When it is nearly dry but still a bit damp, work a small amount of gel or humectant pomade into your hands and then scrunch your hair up. A little goes a long way—if you use too much it will weigh your hair down instead of making it look messy. Finally, spray with hair spray and gently tease your hair.

Ceremony

So now you're all dressed. Put your jewelry on and any temporary tattoos. Choose a symbol that has personal meaning for you.

Choose some music to play. For this glamour you want something with a strong beat. I like trance music, like "Shaman's Breath" by Professor Trance and the Energizers. I also like the CD *Oceania*, which has a track called "Kotahitanga" that is a *haka* (Maori war dance), and *The Gathering* by Inlakesh. You can use rock music. Make sure you choose something empowering that makes you feel strong.

Put the music on and turn it up loud.

INVOCATION

Stand up tall in a warrior stance with your feet apart, knees slightly bent. Close your eyes and hold your arms up toward the sky. Imagine Scathach, the warrior goddess, before you. Call out to her:

Scathach

Goddess of power and might

Fill me with your mighty power

Let your strength radiate through me

Let your confidence fill me

Show me my own power

Let it grow bold and bright

Make my footsteps sure and steady

Scathach

Be with me today

DANCE YOUR POWER

As you feel the power of Scathach fill your body, begin to move to the music. Keep your eyes closed, as it is easier to concentrate. Imagine you are a Celtic warrior whom Scathach has trained for many days and many nights to get into tip-top shape for the task before you.

Close your eyes. Breathe deeply. Breathe in power from the floor, imagining you are pulling strength up from the earth. Hold your arms outstretched again and breathe in, imagining this time you are pulling in strength from the powers of the sun, moon, and stars. Breathe in deeply once more, this time drawing power from the world around you—the trees, the mountains, and your spirit helpers. Feel the power build in your belly. Breathe it in all the way to your stomach region.

Now bring your attention into your body. What part of your body wants to move to the music? Follow your body's whisperings and don't censor yourself with your mind. Just dance. Allow yourself to be free and uninhibited. This is where closing your eyes can help. How does your body want to move? Let the music move through you. Feel your power in your body and dance the dance of a great warrior.

Now imagine the situation where you need power or that has made you mad. Imagine the situation before you and see yourself as Scathach the warrior goddess. Dance the situation as you would like it to be. Keep your eyes closed and stay in your imagination. Pray for help from Scathach. As you dance, see if you get any insights or guidance about the situation. Keep dancing until you do. Then write your insights down in your goddess diary.

Scathach's Tasks for You

- Get some kind of physical exercise every day this week. This may mean going for a walk each morning or going for a run or just putting some loud rock music on the stereo and dancing for fifteen minutes. Before you begin to exercise, close your eyes and visualize Scathach helping you. Say a prayer to her: "Scathach, fill me with your strength, your power, and your courage." Feel the power of this goddess filling you.

- Choose one task that you have been putting off doing because you are too scared to do it. Choose something difficult. This could be anything from confronting a friend about something she did that you didn't like to getting your science project done. Write the date one week from today right here _____. This is the date where you are going to do this hard thing. Each day from now till this date, spend ten minutes each day visualizing yourself doing this hard thing successfully with Scathach's assistance. Ask her for suggestions as to how best to approach the task at hand. Write down any insights in your goddess diary. Keep repeating to yourself: "I can do hard things."

- Look for a magical *symbolic* weapon. No, I do not want you to run to the nearest gun shop and apply for a permit. I don't want you to get any kind of actual weapon at all. What I do want is for you to get something symbolic that can represent your own Gae Bulga. You will know it when you see it. Ask the goddess to bring it to you. Don't be in a hurry to acquire it—it may come as a gift. I was given a tiny pink Swiss pocketknife by a boyfriend once when I was moving away. For years I carried that knife with me wherever I went. Another magical weapon I own is a tiny silver sword on a black velvet choker. I wear this whenever I want to bring out Scathach's powers if I will be facing someone I don't particularly like or trust.

Extra Reading

Read Morgan Llywelyn's *The Red Branch* (Ivy Books, 1990). This is my favorite retelling of the cattle raid of Cooley. You will learn all about Scathach, her sister Ayfa, the great warrior Cuchulain, and Queen Maeve, another famous warrior.

Get a good exercise book or video out of the library, one that is on an exercise you would like to learn.

138

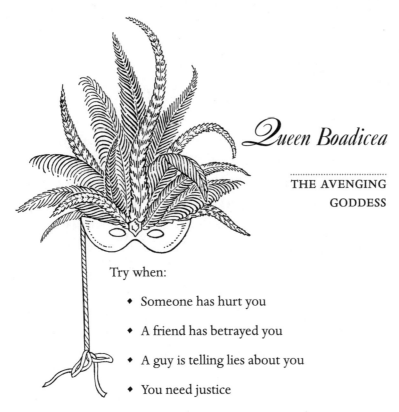

Queen Boadicea

Try when:

* Someone has hurt you

* A friend has betrayed you

* A guy is telling lies about you

* You need justice

* You are dealing with any kind of abuse—
  sexual, physical, emotional, verbal, or mental

Queen Boadicea (pronounced *bo-ah-dee-ka*) is a woman who actually lived a long time ago. Her husband was the king of the Celtic Iceni tribe. When he died, the Romans invaded her lands, tied her up, publicly flogged her, then raped her two young daughters. Queen Boadicea could have let her enemies crush her spirit. Instead she chose to unite as many Celtic tribes as possible and fight back against the Romans.

A warrior woman, Queen Boadicea led the revolt against the Romans. Before each battle she would call on the goddess Andraste (pronounced *ann-drah-stay*) for help. Her animal ally was a hare. Queen Boadicea managed to reclaim Albany, Colchester, and London from the Romans before her death.

Queen Boadicea's Story

Hell hath no fury like a mother scorned

Once upon a time, a long, long time ago, there was a feisty woman with long red hair that fell to her hips, flaming like blood on the tip of a spear. She was tall in stature with glowing green eyes and a voice as loud as a horn at the start of battle on a hot summer's day. This woman was known to all as Boadicea, Celtic Queen of the Iceni. Her husband had just died, leaving her to raise her two teenage daughters and carry on the leadership of their clan. She attacked this task with full gusto, wearing her strength and stubbornness as a shield to counter attacks from those who might wish her harm.

She had one task, and one task only: To hold her tribe together and protect her daughters' rights. This was no easy task, for at that time the Romans were invading Britain and much of the country was in uneasy turmoil. The Romans were known for their brutality; however, they were not counting on Boadicea's ability to fight back.

Now the Romans, in their ignorance, thought a woman ruler was easy prey. "She won't be any trouble to conquer," they mused. "Plus her husband signed over half the ownership of the tribe to our emperor on his deathbed anyway."

When the king's will was read, Boadicea was pained to discover her husband's betrayal. All her life had been devoted to her clan and their welfare. She would not see it go into the Romans' hands. She set about to keep her focus on her task. She was determined her daughters and her people would not fall under Roman rule.

The Romans, however, had other plans. They feared her daughters could marry powerful chiefs from other clans and gain power against them, starting a revolt. They would fix this before it could happen, they decided. So they burst upon the Iceni tribe and raped Boadicea's daughters so that no Celtic man would want them. Then they publicly flogged Queen Boadicea.

Boadicea was beside herself. Within a couple of months, her whole life had turned upside down. "I have lost my husband," she cried. "I have lost half my property to my enemies. I have seen my precious daughters raped by those 'civilized' barbarians. They have whipped me in front of my tribe. If they think I am going to sit quietly at home after such treatment and let them walk all over me, they can think again."

Fueled by her rage, Boadicea gathered her tribe around her. She paid a visit to neighboring clans and called warriors to join her mission.

"We must join forces to fight against the Roman barbarians," she beseeched. "They have stolen our properties, disgraced our daughters, and hurt our people. Let us not sit back and allow one more moment of this crime."

So saying, the finest warriors in the entire south joined Boadicea to fight against the Romans and take back their lands. Boadicea prayed to the battle goddess Andraste for help. "O mighty goddess," she prayed. "You too are a woman like me. Guide my actions, protect my people, lend me your strength, O mighty goddess."

Soon the Romans learned that the south, which they had only recently procured, was in flames. The Queen of the Iceni had risen in revolt.

Orders were sent to the Roman general, Cerealis Petillus, to squash the rebellion. However, by the time Petillus had gathered his soldiers together, Boadicea had marched with her warriors to the city of Colchester and claimed it back from Roman rule.

Boadicea had led her warriors to lie in wait in the woods along the road leading to Colchester. As the Roman legion approached, the Celts ambushed, slashing their enemies to pieces. Next they moved into the town of Colchester, which was the center of Roman government in Britain. Boadicea led her army to the Roman temple dedicated to Claudius before his death. She stared at the hated reminder of the man who had conquered them.

"Down with it!" she cried. And all hell broke out as Boadicea and her band of warriors crushed the building to the ground. Next she turned her fury on the townspeople of Colchester. Some of these people were retired Roman legionnaires; others were Brits with pro-Roman tendencies. "Kill them all!" she entreated. Before long, the lands of Colchester were a bloody mess.

Next Boadicea set out for London. London was founded by the Romans in 43 C.E. and had a population of about 20,000 when Boadicea and her warriors stormed upon it. They burned all the buildings to the ground, and much of the

141

population died under her and her warrior's swords. Boadicea's anger knew no bounds. Nothing was too horrific for the people who had raped her daughters.

Finally Boadicea set out for St. Albans, where again she unleashed her fury. The city of St. Albans reached the same fate as London and Colchester. The basilica, the finely crafted Roman homes, and all public buildings were torched to the ground and the inhabitants slaughtered as Boadicea unleashed her flaming wrath on those who had scorned her.

Boadicea's rebellion was bloody and brutal, but many acts of cruelty had been perpetrated against her people before she fought back. Perhaps Boadicea believed she was fighting for a greater cause of freedom, which made her acts of violence necessary. Remember her lands were under siege by the Romans, who had attacked her first.

Do you think her rage and the way she acted out was merciless or justified?

Know Your Enemies

I used to think everyone was fair, just, and basically good at heart. This was rather a naïve view of the world. While I like to always look for the best in people, I have learned that not everyone plays by the same rules as I do. Some people fight dirty. Some people intend to take things that belong to you. Some people intend to cause others harm.

Recently I was talking with a friend of mine about this. She said when she was younger she used to deliberately set out to hurt other people. I was rather astounded by this, as I like to think people don't intentionally hurt others. "Maybe you just did what you thought was best at the time and didn't know you were going to hurt others by your actions," I suggested.

"Oh no!" she stated. "I knew I was going to hurt people. That was what I wanted to do. I used to sleep with other people's boyfriends and do all kinds of mean stuff."

Her bluntness was refreshingly honest and made me realize that there are people in the world who for whatever reasons seem to get a kick out of causing chaos.

Being discerning is a great asset. Trust your instincts about a person. If you get a weird feeling that someone is not worthy of your trust, go with your gut. Some people are quite predatory. They like to prey on other people and steal things. This can be physical items, like money, possessions, clothing, books, etc. or it can be less tangible things, like boyfriends, best friends, your time, your feelings of self-worth, your energy, or your self-esteem. People who take your self-worth or self-esteem do it by putting you down in subtle or obvious ways by making sarcastic remarks or little digs so you feel "less than" whenever you have been around them. You feel belittled in some way.

People who steal boyfriends or friends do it in a number of ways. They can triangulate by telling your friends something about you that isn't true, or by deliberately exaggerating something you have said to cause trouble in the friendship. I met a girl last year who did this. She would go to one person and say something mean about the other friend and then go to the second friend and say something mean about the first person. She constantly created havoc wherever she went. Another girl I knew was very predatory in her approach. Once she decided what she wanted, she went for it, no matter who was going to be hurt. She seemed to get off on going for other people's boyfriends. She made a habit out of selfishness and stealing. So some people are not going to give a fig about your feelings. You don't have to take it personally. That is just the way some people behave.

How to Spot a Human Predator

These are the people who feed off others. They don't know how to use their own power constructively, or they think they have no power; therefore, they try to steal it from others. Sometimes they do this literally, by taking your boyfriend, your friends, your possessions, or your self-esteem. Sometimes they do this by taking up lots of your precious time by complaining bitterly about their lives. Human predators tend to try to cut you down to make them feel big.

Inside, human predators are generally miserable. Therefore they try to spread their misery around onto everyone else. If you have a human predator in your life, avoid them. Human predators rarely add anything of value to your life. You can

143

have compassion for them; generally human predators' actions are based on envy and fear. However, that doesn't mean you need to be around them.

Here are some common characteristics of human predators:

- They complain a lot about their lives.

- They blame others for their misfortunes.

- They act as if the world owes them a living.

- They "forget" to bring their money when you go out so you end up paying for both of you.

- They flirt with your boyfriend.

- They talk mean about you behind your back.

- They turn up at dinner times so you will feed them.

- They get you to do their homework for them.

- They join your group in projects and never do any of the work.

- They talk about how much better their life will be when they have a boyfriend who has a lot of money and can afford to treat them they way they "deserve" to be treated.

- They belittle you in front of others.

- They steal stuff.

Keep your own behavior impeccable. Don't take what doesn't belong to you. Be trustworthy and honest. Live with integrity and, whenever a human predator comes your way, know that you have the power of the Goddess within you and you don't need to fear anyone.

Preparing for Battle

When you have a battle situation on your hands, like Boadicea, you must take the necessary steps to prepare yourself, mentally and physically. Know that you always have the power of the Goddess on your side.

Some examples of battle:

- Negotiating your wages with an employer

- Settling a conflict with a friend

- Coping with a bully

- Any kind of legal battles

- Dealing with a teacher who has treated you unfairly

- Taking action after any form of sexual abuse

- Guarding your assets (in the form of belongings as well as intangible assets like your time and energy) from those who seek to steal from you

- Standing up for yourself against people who wish to cut you down out of jealousy or insecurity

- Protecting yourself from human predators

- Defending yourself from emotional blackmail, verbal abuse, and any kind of manipulative behavior

Make a Battle Plan

Before a warrior goes into battle, she must assess her weapons and her strengths. What are your weapons? What are your strengths? When I speak of weaponry, I am not talking about physical weapons but rather spiritual weapons. Your weapons can be your focus, your determination, your sense of purpose, and your desire to defend what belongs to you. Your strengths can be your ability to stay positive under extreme pressure, your ability to stand up for yourself, and your desire to right a wrong.

What is the battle at hand? What is it that you are fighting for?

Get clear in your mind the desired outcome. See yourself as victorious.

Gather Your Allies

Who are the people you can call on for help? Do you have friends who will support you and go forth with you on your cause? Who are the people you know who will cut you down or belittle you? Make sure you keep your plans to yourself or only share them with people who will help you.

Enlist the Help of Spiritual Allies

Who are the beings in the spirit world you can call on for help? Like Queen Boadicea, you can call on the goddess Andraste for help. Her name means "victorious" or "invincible." She is a Celtic battle goddess. Talk to her, woman to woman, like Boadicea did before each battle. Ask for her protection and guidance. Ask her to inspire you with creative ideas of how to reach your desired outcome.

You can call on Boadicea for help, too. Have a conversation with her in your imagination. All you have to do is close your eyes and see a mental picture of Queen Boadicea. Imagine her with her flaming red hair down to her hips, wearing a long green tartan dress, belted at the waist with a gold belt. Around her neck is a gold torque and around her head is a golden headband inscribed with magical Celtic symbols. She carries a long spear in her arms and her golden cloak is fastened at the neck with a beautiful Celtic brooch. She is wise in the ways of battle. She will be your protector and spiritual mentor. Ask her advice. Say her name three times in your imagination, and then ask her what suggestions she has for you. She will show you in pictures what you can do, or tell you in words. Write down what she says.

Take Guided Action

Pray to Boadicea to help you come up with constructive actions that will move you forward in your quest. Make a list of actions you can take. Pray for courage and strength to carry them out.

Fight with All Your Might

Once you have decided to take up your cause, give it your all. Let nothing or no one stand in your way. Don't think about failing, think about achieving the best possible outcome for all concerned.

....

Goddess Workout

Write down a situation that has been troubling you where you have not been standing up for your rights.

Write down your strengths.

List your weapons.

Who are your allies?

Who are the people you can't trust, the ones who are not on your side?

Who are the people who actually wish you harm?

Write a battle plan for dealing with this situation.

What guided action can you take?

Encountering a Surprise Attack

You can't always control every situation but you can always control how you react. You can take charge of the situation. You can take control of your life. You're in charge of your life, your thoughts, and your actions. So even if someone knocks the breath out of you metaphorically by doing something that hurts you, you can empower yourself by acting in a way that moves you forward instead of sending your life into a tailspin.

If a situation arises where you are at the mercy of another person's mean-spiritedness, gather your thoughts together. Assess the situation objectively. What damage has been done thus far? What can you do to prevent further damage? What steps do you need to take to care for yourself?

Use the "preparing for battle" strategy to remain centered in your power and pray to Queen Boadicea for help. See yourself emerging victorious from the situation. Know that no matter how hurt or angry you may feel today at being treated unjustly, you will not only survive, but thrive. Keep your focus on the future and your desired outcome. Know that the Goddess will support you in all your endeavors.

Many times when people get treated unfairly by others, they react in fear, which drains their power away. Don't let yourself get caught in the net of imagining the worst possible scenario. Know that the Goddess is your true source of all love, all money, all resources, and everything you could possibly need. People, places, and things are not your true sources—they are just the avenues through which the Goddess can give you those things. If something is taken from you, then something better will be given in return. Put your faith in the Goddess and know that nothing can destroy you.

Fight for What Is Rightfully Yours

There will be times when you will have to fight for your rights. This is part of knowing your true worth. I used to hate any kind of confrontation. I wanted everyone to like me, and my way of ensuring that was to be a people pleaser, always putting others' needs before my own. Well, not everyone is going to like you anyway, so you may as well get used to that idea, and people respect others who set boundaries and walk all over those who don't. Plus, if you don't stand up for yourself, no one else will.

Use Your Anger as Fuel

Anger is a wonderful weapon to fuel your battles. I am not talking about emotionally throwing up over people here. I am talking about channeling your anger into appropriate action to ensure fairness ensues. You can use your anger to effect great change in the world. You can join a group for a cause that you think is worthwhile, or you can use your anger at being mistreated to ensure you get fairly treated in the future. You can set boundaries with people and make sure they treat you and your belongings with respect. Treat yourself as you would a precious object. Once you start treating yourself that way, others will, too. Anger is a call to action.

149

Call on the Power of Tribal Ancestors

Whenever I have to face a situation that I find daunting, I call on the power of my Maori and Celtic warrior ancestors. You don't have to be Maori or Celtic to do this. Simply ask for a band of Celtic warriors to come to your side. Imagine 10,000 warriors standing behind you. Imagine Boadicea standing before you, invoking the power of Andraste and leading you into battle. When you feel the presence of 10,000 warriors behind you, it is hard to feel scared about something!

Weave a Lorica

A lorica is a magical Celtic prayer that the Celts would weave around themselves as a spiritual breastplate for power and protection. Words were sacred to the Celts and had great power.

Probably the most famous lorica is "St. Patrick's Breastplate." In this prayer, which was written as the Celtic lands were becoming Christianized, St. Patrick invoked the powers of nature, God, and Christ to protect him from those who wished him ill. The first part of the prayer goes like this:

I arm myself today with the might of heaven:

The rays of the sun

The beams of the moon

The glory of fire

The speed of wind

The depth of sea

The stability of earth

The hardness of rock . . .

You can write your own lorica using powers that have meaning for you. Here is one I wrote that you can use as a model:

I gird myself today with the power of the Goddess:

The strength of the sun

The beauty of the stars

The magic of the moon

The spear of Boadicea

The sword of Scathach

The shield of Andraste

The stone of truth and destiny.

I arm myself today with the mighty power of the universe:

May the Goddess's wisdom guide me

May the Goddess's love empower me

May the Goddess's strength protect me

From any who wish me harm

I weave a web of power and protection

Above me and below me

Around me and within me

From my feet to my fingertips

The power of the Goddess

Surrounds and protects me

Alone and with others

And so it is

....

Goddess Workout

Write your own lorica, calling on the powers of nature, the powers of the planets, the powers of the Goddess, and any other powers that have meaning to you.

Creating a Shield of Goddesses for Protection

Whenever you are afraid, you can create a shield of warrior goddesses around your self, your home, and your loved ones. Simply close your eyes and say:

A goddess before me, a goddess behind me

A goddess at my right, a goddess at my left

A goddess above me, a goddess below me

I am surrounded and protected

By the power of the Goddess now

See the circle of goddesses around you, moving with you. Do this before any situation where you feel afraid, like if you are at home alone or traveling. If you unexpectedly bump into someone you don't like, keep doing this, too, to "keep your shields up."

Claiming Your Sovereignty—Celtic Queens and Their Rights

Sovereignty was very important to Celtic peoples. And a queen had even more value than the king, for it was the queen who carried the mantle of sovereignty and could bestow it upon the king. Unless the queen granted sovereignty, the king was unable to rule. Now there were three tasks that the queen must undertake to ensure her sovereignty. The first was to know her true worth, the second was to pick a mate without a blemish—or, in other words, a mate worthy of her—and the third was to know what was worth fighting for and what wasn't.

152

Goddess Workout

What is your true worth?

Who are your true friends—the ones who share the same values as you and treat you with respect?

What in your life is worth fighting for?

What isn't worth fighting over?

Queen Boadicea's Glamour

- Two small hair braids to weave magic in your hair

- A cloak or shawl

- A magical hair band

- A golden choker

- A long skirt

- Her makeup is clean but strong

Makeup

Put a light foundation over your face. Darken your eyebrows with a brown brow pencil. Line your eyes with a silver eye pencil. Use a teal-green cream eye shadow all over your eyelids. Apply a gold shadow across your brow bone. Use a light-brown cream blush to bring out your cheekbones. Gloss your lips with a berry lipstick.

Clothing

Try a long green dress or a tartan skirt with a tank top. Wrap a shawl around your shoulders and secure it with a pretty pin. If you have a Celtic brooch, so much the better. Find a belt that you can charge with magical properties. You can make your own, if you are skilled at leather work, and engrave Celtic symbols into it. If you can't make your own, buy a belt that represents Boadicea to you: a sparkly gold one or a sparkly red or green one are all good Celtic colors. On the inside of the belt draw Celtic symbols with a permanent marker. As you draw them, pray to Boadicea to charge the belt with magical powers of protection so whenever you wear it you are divinely guided.

Queen Boadicea wore a golden torque around her neck. Find a choker or golden necklace that you can wear as a symbol of your goddess power.

Hairstyle

In Celtic times women would weave magical spells into their hair by praying as they braided it. When you get up in the morning, you can weave magic into your day by braiding your hair and praying as you braid it. What would you like to weave into your day today? Whatever you choose, focus on it coming into your life as you braid your hair. Say a prayer such as: "I weave beauty and love into my day today." Repeat the prayer until your hair is completely braided.

One way Celtic women would wear their hair was by braiding two little braids down the sides of their faces and letting the rest of their hair flow loosely down their backs. You can do this, or if your hair is short you can attach tiny hair braids on clips from an accessories store such as Claire's.

Find a hair band and wrap it around your forehead. I have a beautiful Celtic one that I bought from a metaphysical bookstore. Many metaphysical bookstores carry Celtic jewelry. Another alternative is to wear a fun crown from a party store.

Ceremony

Have a shower and wash any fears down the drain. Visualize all your fears falling from your body right down the drainpipe. Wash your hair and wash out all your fear. Finish with a cool rinse.

Put on your makeup and spray yourself with a woodsy fragrance, invoking the power of the Celtic warriors as you do so.

Get dressed in your Queen Boadicea outfit. As you put on your shawl, imagine you are wrapping the protection and strength of the goddess around you. Fasten your brooch to the shawl and hold your head up high. Now you are ready to put on your hair band. As you put the hair band on, imagine you are being crowned with your sovereignty. You are the Queen of Justice and you will stand up for yourself.

Get your lorica out and put on some music that makes you feel strong. Find jewelry that is precious to you, perhaps jewelry that you have been given as a present by your grandparents, parents, or special friends. You can also wear a low necklace that comes down to your heart to wear as a shield and protect your heart from hurt. Another idea is to get a small round mirror from a craft store and stick it to your heart facing outwards with makeup glue. This way anyone who sends you "looks that can kill" will have their intentions reflected right back at them.

Close your eyes and invoke the power of Boadicea. Imagine her standing right in front of you, about ten feet tall. Her eyes are fierce, her hair flaming down her back. She holds the Spear of Justice in her hands. Now feel Queen Boadicea's power surging through you. Her strength courses through your veins. You feel invincible, powerful, and victorious in the face of your enemies. Expand your aura so you can see it in your imagination about ten feet tall. Pretend you, too, are holding the Spear of Justice in your hands. With your intent, you can focus your spear-like will and produce the desired outcome to protect your sovereignty and reign victorious. Pray:

Boadicea, goddess of the mighty battle

Protect me from my enemies

Let your courage be my courage

Let your strength be my strength

Guide me from all who wish me ill

Let me see with the eyes of the Goddess

Let me speak with the words of the Goddess

Let me act with the actions of the Goddess

I weave a web of strength, courage, and faith

Around myself now in your name

Now read your lorica and see in your imagination the most beautiful breastplate you have ever seen forming around your torso. No one can hurt you, for you are divinely protected. You go forth into the world with confidence and power from the Goddess.

Queen Boadicea's Tasks for You

- Choose one situation this week that has been making you angry or irritated. What are you going to do about it? Pray to Boadicea for help. Then take three tiny steps toward resolving the situation.

- Who in your life makes you the maddest? What is it that this person does that causes you to feel so angry? How do you normally react to this person? Change your reactions and see if this changes the situation.

- Know your true worth. What is your true worth? How do you let people treat you? You are a precious daughter of the Goddess. Do you act like this or do you cower with fear in front of others? Imagine you are a daughter of the Goddess and wear your royalty with pride.

- For one day, dress up as Queen Boadicea and go out into the world acting as the royal Queen. How does it feel to be queen for a day?

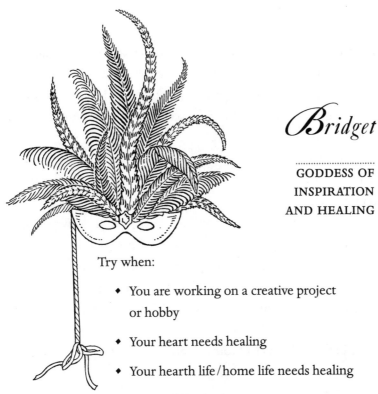

Bridget

....

**GODDESS OF
INSPIRATION
AND HEALING**

Try when:

• You are working on a creative project
  or hobby

• Your heart needs healing

• Your hearth life / home life needs healing

• You need inspiration

Bridget (pronounced *bridge-it*) is another woman who really
lived. Actually there are two Bridgets—the first was the goddess from ancient Celtic mythology, the second was a woman
who lived from A.D. 452 to A.D. 524. She became Saint Bridget
in the Catholic Church. There are many similarities between
the goddess and the saint, and some people believe that St.
Bridget's life was touched by the goddess Bridget.

In this chapter you will meet both Bridget the Celtic goddess and Bridget the woman. Bridget the Celtic goddess is
goddess of poetry, healing, and smithcrafts. She is a fire goddess of the home and of crafts that use fire, like silversmithing
or blacksmithing. She is the Great Goddess of the heart.
When you have no fiery passion in your heart, she will kindle
the fire for you so you regain your spark and enthusiasm for
life.

The other Bridget you will meet in this chapter is Bridget of Kildare, who was closely related to the earlier Celtic goddess who shared her name; indeed, they share many qualities. Bridget's life was touched by divine fire and many of her stories, as with the earlier goddess, have a strong association with fire. Fire was central to daily life for the Celtic people.

Bridget became a Mother Abbess when she was only twenty-two years old. She was often called "Mary of the Celts." She could cure sick people who were thought to be incurable. Even her shadow was so powerful that it could heal, too. Wherever she went, things prospered tenfold: food, drink, livestock, vegetables, everything! So there would always be plenty in her presence. People loved having Bridget around because they knew they were always assured of prosperity.

When you call on Bridget, she will work miracles in your life. She will cause the things you love to multiply and prosper. You will have way more than you need.

Bridget can also help you to heal a broken heart. She cures the inconsolable. She is truly a compassionate, loving, mother goddess.

Bridget's Story

Bridget, the miracle worker

Once upon a time, a long, long time ago, there was a beautiful young maiden named Bridget who lived with her mother, raising cattle.

Bridget was as fiery as a goddess with her long golden hair that flashed brilliantly around her head and upper body like a halo of golden sunshine. Even her face seemed to shine with the radiance of a summer's day. Everywhere she went, people basked in the warmth of her smile and the kindness of her heart.

One day a young man of the village who had long held a flame for Bridget in his heart came to visit her. "Bridget," he declared, "make me the happiest man in the village and become my bride." But Bridget gently refused, saying, "I cannot marry anyone, for I have important work to do in the world and my work must always come first."

Bridget blazed with the passion of inner conviction, and nothing and no one could sway her from her path. One day she told her mother, "Mother, I intend to become a nun. I have seen that I have a lot of work to do in the world and I must begin it now." So off Bridget went to join the order of nuns at Telch Mide.

When she arrived, Bishop Mel greeted her at the door. The bishop just about fell over when he set eyes on the young woman before him. That very night, he had dreamed of the mother of God, and in his dream her face was exactly the same as the girl before him. From this point on, Bridget was often referred to as "Mary of the Gaels/Celts."

Bridget loved her life in the holy order. Each prayer, each recital of the rosary she performed with sacred devotion. And before long it was time for Bridget to take her vows along with the other novices.

The girls were greatly excited to dedicate their lives to the service of God. They understood the magnitude of such a decision and wore the responsibility as a cloak of great honor. One by one, the young girls moved toward the prelate and took their vows.

When it was Bridget's turn, the prelate accidentally read out the wrong words. Instead of the words to proclaim her as a nun, he said the words to proclaim her an Abbess—Mother Superior!

The order was in an uproar. The elders began to protest vehemently that the words be revoked. "We cannot have this!" they cried. "Why, she is too young to hold such an honored position. She is barely twenty-two!" While the uproar continued, Bishop Mel looked toward Bridget. "Quiet!" he commanded. "Quickly, look and see!" All heads turned toward Bridget, and were amazed to see a flame of fire surrounding her. The elders stood back in awe and Bishop Mel announced, "This is a sign from God. Bridget has been chosen by Him to be the Mother Abbess." And so it was that Bridget became an abbess at the tender age of twenty-two!

Bridget soon became known as a miracle worker. People spoke about how she could cure lepers and give blind people sight. She could put her hands over a broken bone and mend it back together. Word quickly spread throughout the entire land of her amazing abilities, and people flocked to see her. One day a little boy who was mute came to see her. Bridget asked him a question and immediately he began to speak.

Even her shadow could heal others, so powerful was her healing gift. When she lay her hands over milk or water and said a blessing, the liquid would bring miracles to those who drank it.

Like King Midas, Bridget had the golden touch. Whatever she touched increased. Bridget would visit communities whose food supplies were dwindling and wherever she went everything would multiply. There would be plenty of food to eat and ale to drink. Even the sheep and cattle and crops would multiply.

As more and more people came to see her to be healed, to hear her teachings, or just to bask in her presence, Bridget realized she needed her own abbey: a center where people could visit for healings or teachings.

So off she went, in search of a site to build such a center. One day she was stopped in the middle of a road by a caravan of carts all overflowing with wood which was to be taken to the great chief Aillil who lived near Kildare in Leinster. Bridget went to see Aillil and asked him, "May I use some of your wood to build an abbey?"

Aillil glared down at the young woman and said, "I will not even give you one stick!"

At the moment he spoke, all the carts came to a standstill and would not budge. Indeed, it seemed as if they were rooted to the spot by a mysterious force. Aillil's men tried using brute force to get the carts moving again, but to no avail. Nothing moved.

Finally Aillil bowed before Bridget and said, "Mistress, it would seem a higher authority than mine has declared this wood for your use. Take whatever you need."

So Bridget built her abbey at Kildare on land that was once a ceremonial ground for the ancient Druids. On the day the building was complete, Bridget stood in front of the main hearth and lit the fire. As she did so, she prayed out loud: "May this light burn forever in the world and may it never be allowed to go out."

And today the flame of Bridget still burns brightly.

The Goddess Bridget

In Celtic times, before Christianity, the goddess Bridget was worshipped all over Europe. She was one of the most important goddesses in the Celtic tradition. A fire goddess, she was the goddess of healing, inspiration, and smithcraft. She was a triple goddess, as the following verse shows her threefold nature and how each of her aspects is associated with fire (author unknown):

Fire in the forge that shapes and tempers

Fire in the cauldron that nourishes and heals

Fire in the head that incites and inspires

Bridget was the daughter of the Celtic god Dagda, one of the Tuatha de Dannan. She protected women during childbirth and many prayers were uttered to her by pregnant women. An ancient Celtic custom was for pregnant women to say a prayer at a spring to Bridget, and make a small fire in her honor. Many springs in Ireland are still sacred to Bridget. Saint Bridget is also known for her holy water and people will make pilgrimages to the springs to gather water in her name and use it for healing and blessings.

Bridget's festival is on February 1, and is also known as Imbolc or Candlemas. This is one of the great Celtic festivals. There are eight in the year and they are all based on the solar calendar. Imbolc is a fertility festival, which celebrates the lactation of ewes and the birth of livestock. Bridget was especially concerned about the welfare of livestock and cattle.

Bridget was represented by a doll on her feast day. Young girls dressed in white carried Bridget dolls (also called corn dollies) made out of corn. People would give gifts of food to the goddess doll to receive her blessing for a bountiful summer. Young girls would partake in a special feast for the Goddess, which took place in a locked room. After a while, the boys of the community could join in the feasting after they had asked for permission to enter so they, too, could worship Bridget.

One custom held on February 1 in honor of Bridget is a spring cleaning. The house is cleaned from top to bottom, and the women call out to the Goddess to welcome her. The oldest woman of the house represents the Goddess in her crone aspect and she puts out the fire in the hearth. Then the fireplace is cleaned out. The youngest girl present represents the Goddess in her maiden phase. She enters the house through the front door carrying a candle in honor of Bridget. The girl is traditionally dressed in white and wears a crown of lit candles. The young girl re-lights the fire in the hearth. This celebrates the Goddess in her maiden phase for the oncoming spring where everything old is new again. The Earth Mother is re-born once more into the maiden of spring.

162

....

Goddess Workout

Clean out your bedroom. Throw or give away everything you no longer use or need. Get rid of the old to make room for the new. Give the floors a good sweep. Then light a candle in honor of Bridget.

Say a prayer over the flame: "Goddess Bridget, I ask your blessing on my life. May it be filled to overflowing with goodness and love. May you bring prosperity and happiness to me. May your warmth light my home and my heart. Thank you, dear Goddess."

The Importance of Fire in Celtic Tradition

Fire was used for heating, cooking, cleaning, washing, and making crafts, and it was central to Celtic life. The fire was always placed in the center of the home.

Fire was of utmost importance in Celtic times. Most houses were either round or oblong in shape. Right in the middle of the home was the cauldron, which was heated by a huge fire. There was usually only one room in Celtic homes. Everybody ate, slept, cooked, and did their chores in the same room. There wasn't much furniture in the houses—no chairs for sitting on, but rather a bench along the walls made from packed earth where people would sleep and sit to eat.

A huge cauldron would hang by iron chains from the ceiling over the hearth. The hearth was the heart of the family's home. Many cold, dark winter nights were warmed by the hearth fire. It provided heat for cooking. Huge quantities of meat would boil in the cauldron above the hearthstones. The fire gave off light, too, which was important, as there were no windows in the home.

Fire was used in metalworking and blacksmithing. Much of the Celts' wealth came from their excellence in metalwork. They were famous for their intricate designs. Bronze was used to make jewelry, household implements, and to decorate their weapons. Iron was used to make tools and weapons. Metalworkers were honored in Celtic society and held a position of respect.

163

The Flame of Kildare—It Still Burns Today

Today there are still orders devoted to keeping the flame of Bridget burning. You can check out the website http://www.ordbrighideach.org to learn about the flamekeepers for the Ord Brighideach.

The flamekeepers are voluntary members from all over the world. Each flame keeper is assigned a day on a cycle of twenty-two days to guard the flame. The Celtic day began at sunset and finished the following sunset, which is the day you would watch the flame, unlike our modern days, which begin at 12 A.M. until the following 12 A.M.

Members of the order have a candle that was lit from the original hearth fire at Kildare. When it is your turn, you light your candle and keep it burning until your shift is over. If the candle burns down, you must light another candle from the flame before the lit candle is extinguished. Each order member says a prayer of commitment to the flame on their first shift. Members make up their own prayers that have a special meaning to them.

There are over 350 members in the Ord Brighideach. The website is a great place to visit to read poetry and stories about Bridget that members have contributed.

Bridget and Mary

Bridget was often called Mary of the Celts. She has many qualities of Mother Mary from the Christian faith, who may be considered a deity according to our definition of a goddess. Even though Christians don't define Mary as a goddess, she is a greatly adored woman, which—according to the dictionary—is status enough for her to be considered a goddess. Bridget, like Mary, was a woman of great compassion. She was also an intercessor between people and God. Both women were totally devoted in their service to God.

If you feel the need for support or unconditional love, you can turn to Mary or Bridget. They will listen. They will hold your heart in their hands and comfort you in times of great sorrow or despair.

Light a Candle, Talk to Bridget

The next time you have a problem or your heart feels heavy, get a candle—perhaps a Roman Catholic candle with a picture of Mary on it, or a yellow candle, as Bridget is often associated with gold, and then sit down and light the candle. Tell Bridget exactly what is on your heart. Pour out all your sorrows, your heartaches, tell her everything that is troubling you. Picture her as a kind mother who wants what is best for you. Rub your hands together to heat them and then place them over your heart and visualize your hands as the hands of Bridget. Feel the warmth of her love healing your heart.

Rekindling Your Hearth Fire at Home and In Your Heart

If you live in a home where there is not much harmony, there is a lot you can do to improve things. First, ask Bridget for help. Keep a candle burning in her honor in your bedroom—make sure you use either a candle in a glass container and away from curtains or anything flammable. Only have the flame going while you are in the room.

To brighten the energy in your home, open the windows and front door once a day for twenty minutes. This will help to keep the air fresh and remove any negative energy left over from arguments. Put some fresh flowers on the table in one of the rooms. Play soothing music—you could leave the radio on the classical station playing while everyone is out. This will definitely help to change the vibration of the home.

When you go to bed at night and before you get out of bed in the morning, visualize everyone in your house. Send them love one by one. Imagine them surrounded in a giant egg of golden light. Ask Bridget to help you heal the atmosphere in your home and to rekindle the hearth fire. Imagine Bridget walking through your house holding a magical candle. She goes from room to room, clearing the air from all unkind words that have been uttered, all bad feelings, all meanness and hurt. She sprinkles golden Celtic fairy dust everywhere, which has a healing effect on all the people in your home.

Do what you can at home to promote a feeling of happiness. Even if things are very miserable, *you* don't need to be miserable. Make your own private space a place that brings you comfort. Hang up posters that brighten your mood. Try not to react to family members with bad feelings. Even if you feel mad at someone, consider what you will say. When you lash out in anger, your words have a destructive effect. You can set boundaries with people without putting a dagger in their sides.

Visualize a bright golden aura surrounding you for protection before you enter your house. Ask the angels of Bridget to form a circle of love and protection around your home. Ask them to remove any negative energy, too, and to infuse your home with love.

Healing Your Heart: A Sacred Heart Meditation

If your heart has been hurt, Bridget is a great goddess to go to for healing. Many people think if their heart has been broken it will take ages to mend. Actually this is not the case at all. Your heart is very, very strong. It begins mending as soon as someone hurts it, just as a wound or injury begins to heal as soon as it has happened. There are many things you can do, though, to help with the healing process. One is this sacred heart meditation.

Stand with your arms outstretched and your feet about shoulder-width apart. Close your eyes.

See Bridget standing in front of you with a flame of fire upon her head and extending from her hands. Her whole body radiates with a golden glow.

Breathe in very deeply. Feel the air fill your lungs and move all the way down to your toes.

Now imagine Bridget putting her hands on your heart. She is sending her healing love into your heart to make it whole again. Keep breathing deeply and breathe this love into your entire body.

Do this for about five minutes.

Then bring your hands into a prayer position and say thank you to Bridget.

Try not to talk too much about whatever it was that caused you pain. The more you talk about painful stuff, the more you keep it alive. Instead, focus on what is good in your life and talk about that. When you focus on a painful event you keep reliving it in your mind over and over. Plus your body cannot distinguish between things you vividly imagine and things that are really happening. This keeps the pain stuck around you. Ask Bridget to help you cultivate joy in your life. Look for simple things to do that bring you joy.

If you find yourself stuck in the pain or sadness of a past event, do something physical to move the energy out. Clap your hands vigorously for a minute, do ten jumping jacks, sing nursery songs at the top of your lungs. It doesn't matter what you do so long as you do something to break the pattern of pain.

Remember, hearts have an amazing ability to heal.

Write a Heart Cluster Poem

This is how to write a poem with the help of Bridget, a poem from your heart, using heart clusters.

If you have a fireplace you can do this in the winter with a real fire; otherwise, just use a candle.

One Celtic custom was to use fire as a divination tool. On the days of the great solar festivals, like Imbolc, Druids (the Celtic priests and priestesses) could look into the bonfires and divine the future. You can use the power of fire, too, to divine your own future.

Wait for the Celtic day to begin. Remember, the new day starts at sunset. So start this practice at sunset, too. Light a fire in the fireplace or light a candle and gaze at the flames. Don't have any other lights on. Keep gazing for at least twenty minutes. Ask Bridget to anoint you with the flame of inspiration. Squint your eyes and stare into the fire—see if you can make out any images. Talk to the fire. Ask it to inspire you with fire in your head.

Then pick up a piece of paper and start making notes. Just write down words randomly. Circle the words and write down more words that come to mind. Do this until you get the urge to start writing sentences.

Begin to write a poem. Write any kind of poem—a love poem, a silly poem, a poem about injustices or hurts you have suffered. Poetry was a sacred art form in Celtic times. Bards would study and memorize poems for nine years. They were the record keepers of Celtic history. Poems can help you make a statement about something that hurts you or heals you or interests you. Write your poem out on a clean sheet of paper and decorate it with little drawings.

Ceremony to Create Prosperity

Bridget is the goddess of prosperity and miracles. Whatever she touches increases. You can ask her for a miracle in your life whenever you need one. If you want more prosperity in your life, you need to start thinking of yourself as prosperous. See yourself as being a part of the universe's unlimited resources. See great things flowing toward you. Go for a walk and notice the abundance in nature—zillions of stars in the sky, trillions of blades of grass on the ground. Know that it is your birthright to be prosperous.

Make a treasure map of what you would like in your life.

Get a large sheet of paper.

Stick your photo in the middle. Then look through magazines and find pictures of things you would like to become or to have in your life. Make it as realistic as possible. Dream big. If you would like to travel to far-off places, then look for pictures of locales you would like to visit. If you would like to become a famous author, then stick pictures of books on your treasure map and write your name underneath them. If you would like a boyfriend, then find a picture of a guy who looks like someone you would like to go out with.

Practice seeing yourself having and being all the things in your treasure map. Write positive statements on your map, like "This is me with my new boyfriend" or "Here I am visiting the pyramids in Egypt."

Once the map is finished, say a prayer to Bridget:

Goddess Bridget

Mother of miracles

Patron lady of prosperity

I ask you to bless this map of my life

Show me the steps I need to take to get there

Illuminate my path

Bring to me those who can help me fulfill my dreams

As you fulfilled yours

And so might it be

Light a green candle to attract prosperity into your life and hang your map on your bedroom wall or inside your locker.

Mothering the Motherless

If you don't have a mother or your mother is emotionally or physically absent a lot, Bridget can be your surrogate mother. Find a small picture that looks like her to you. You could get a card of Saint Bridget from a Roman Catholic supply store. Carry the card around with you. Talk to the picture as you would to a real mother. Imagine her talking back to you. When you have problems or need some motherly advice, do the "light a candle" exercise in this chapter.

Even though you may not have a mother in the physical world, you do have a mother in the spiritual realms. The Goddess is the divine mother of all, and she is always ready and willing to listen to you and to offer her loving advice. When you have a crappy day, lie down on your bed and imagine the Goddess wrapping her arms around you, comforting you and holding you in love.

I have done this exercise often. My mother died when I was twenty-one and there have been many times when I have turned to the Goddess when I missed my mother. Sometimes the Goddess has come to me before I have even had a chance to ask her to! After the birth of my first son, I was in a lot of pain one night. I felt utterly wretched. I was so exhausted and my C-section wound was hurting. In my room I saw the Goddess propped up on the bed beside me. Her aura filled the entire room with a golden glow. I immediately felt at peace and comforted. You can imagine her with you whenever you want.

If you feel misunderstood by your own mother, pray to Bridget for help. Ask her to heal the rift between you and your mother so you can have a good relationship with her. Ask Bridget what you need to do to help your mother understand you.

Bridget's Glamour

- Apricot lipstick

- Red and gold ribbons in your hair

- Sparkly red nail polish

- A heart-shaped necklace

- A golden locket

- Yellow candle

- Milk with honey and cinnamon—Bridget's magic milk recipe

- Her makeup is warm and enticing. She is the golden girl of the Celts. Everything about her looks rich and lavish and emphasizes warmth.

Makeup

This is a great glamour for during the summer. Think golden girl or California beach bum. Even though Bridget's skin was probably quite pale, she had a rosy glow.

Use a tinted moisturizer to give your skin a golden sheen. Then apply a sparkly green pencil eyeliner around your eyes. Across your brow bone apply a gold cream eye shadow. On the inner corner apply a bright green cream eye shadow, on the outer corner apply a bright blue and then in the middle apply pink. Coat your lashes with lots of black mascara.

Use a peach blush on your cheeks and an apricot lip gloss on your lips.

Clothing

If you want to be traditionally Celtic, wear a long, green, velvet dress. Otherwise, a more modern approach will suffice. You can try a pair of cargo pants and a green T-shirt—think of yourself as a warrior for love. You could try a floral sundress—think of yourself as expressing the abundance of Bridget.

Hairstyle

Wash your hair and scrunch it dry so it has a tousled just-got-out-of-bed look. Try tying little gold and red ribbons through it. You can spray some golden glitter in it, too, for a sparkly effect.

Ceremony

When you are dressed as Bridget, say an invocation to allow her energy to enter you:

Goddess Bridget

Bright lady

Illumined one

Fill me with your radiance

Inspire me with fire in my head

Fire in my heart

And fire in my soul

Now see yourself as totally on fire for life. If there is an issue that you feel enflamed about, take some action on it. Write a letter to a government representative explaining your ideals. Send a small donation to a charity that you like. Take a homeless person something to eat—do this with an adult. Be kind to someone at school that others pick on. This glamour is all about taking action to make a difference in the world, just like Bridget did.

See Bridget's healing energy flowing through you and use it today to make a difference. Make your world a little brighter, and the lives of those around you a little brighter, too.

Bridget's Tasks for You

- Write yourself a love letter. Start it out "Dear _____, these are all the things I love about you . . ." Write whatever you can think of, big and small. Write about your accomplishments that you are proud of big and small. Whenever you feel down about yourself, pull this letter out and read it.

- Write Bridget a letter telling her about your heart's desires. Write all the things you would like to have in your life. Remember, she is the goddess of miracles and prosperity, and nothing is impossible to her.

- What kind of fire brightens your life? Where is your inner fire? How do you use it? Write ways you can bring more warmth and love into your life and then do one thing off your list.

- Dress as Bridget one day this week and go out into the world as her. How does it feel to be the goddess of healing and inspiration? Write about your experiences in your goddess journal.

Radiate your goddess power today

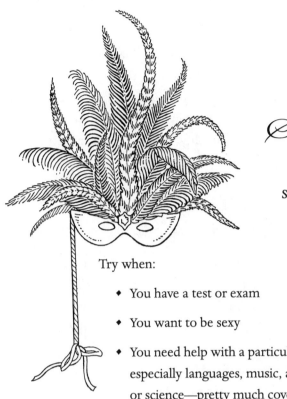

Sarasvati

....

**GODDESS OF
SCHOOLWORK,
MUSIC, AND
SENSUALITY**

Try when:

- You have a test or exam

- You want to be sexy

- You need help with a particular subject,
  especially languages, music, arts, math,
  or science—pretty much covers it all,
  doesn't it!

- You have to write a paper

- You want inspiration with any creative
  endeavor

Sarasvati (pronounced *sa-ra-svah-tee*) is the Hindu goddess of
learning, inspiration, and music. She was renowned for her
beauty and grace. Sarasvati is the queen of knowledge and education who invented the sacred Sanskrit alphabet and mathe-
matics. Today students in India ask her for help with their
exams.

Sarasvati is the beautiful wife of the creator god Brahma.
She became the mother of the universe. Brahma taught Sarasvati how to create things of great beauty. She was given the

power to create whatever Brahma dreamed up in his head. She can help you create whatever you dream up in your head, too.

She is the goddess of music, creative arts, language, learning, science, and sensuality. She receives all words just as the ocean receives all streams. Words flow to her and from her, as do creativity and sensuality. Whenever you are stuck for words, call on Sarasvati to flow through you and inspire your speech.

Sarasvati's Story

How Sarasvati bestowed the gift of love

Once upon a time, a long, long time ago, there was a beautiful goddess named Sarasvati. Her skin was pale and luminous and glowed more powerfully than the sheen of a million moons rising into the darkening sky. Her hair was long and dark, framing her face like the sky at midnight. Her eyes were deep pools of ebony glistening with the dew of compassion.

Sarasvati was so beautiful that her husband Brahma grew five heads just so he could see her from every angle when she was around him. Sarasvati had four arms that represent the four directions. Her front arms relate to the physical, manifest world and her back arms to the spiritual realms. Sarasvati can reach into the spiritual world and manifest whatever she needs in the physical world. She is constantly bringing forth dreams, goals, and visions from the spiritual imagination into physical reality.

With one of her right arms she holds out a flower to her husband, expressing her love and devotion to him. With her other right arm she holds a book made from palm leaves, which shows her love of learning. It was she who invented the Devanagari alphabet. In one left hand she holds a string of beads like a rosary, which symbolizes the need to focus your spiritual power to make your dreams come true, and in her other left hand she holds a small drum.

Sometimes Sarasvati is pictured sitting on a beautiful lotus playing a vina, an Indian lute, which shows her great love of music. Her name means "flowing one" and in India there is a river named for Sarasvati that flows from the Himalayan mountains.

The Story of Sarasvati and Savitri

Once upon a time, a long, long time ago, there was a brave king named Lord of Horses. The king and his wife longed for children; however, none came. So every day the king said prayers to Sarasvati and made offerings to her.

One day Sarasvati appeared before the king and said, "For eighteen years you have honored me with your devotion. Ask what you wish of me."

"Beloved Goddess," said the king, "my wife and I wish to bear sons who will be an honor to our people."

Sarasvati replied, "I cannot gift you with sons; however, I will gift you with a daughter who will be a means to the wish you requested."

And with that said, Sarasvati vanished. Nine months later, the queen bore a daughter who was named Savitri in honor of the Goddess.

And as the young girl grew, she was as beautiful and as gracious as the Goddess herself. Wherever she went, people would say, "There goes the Goddess."

Savitri desired a boyfriend, but the young men were daunted by her brilliance, her beauty, and her incredible shining spirit.

One day her father found her crying and asked, "Tell me, my Savitri, whatever is the matter?"

"Oh, father," she replied, "I long for a husband, a companion like the other girls in the village. I, too, wish for someone to share my heart with."

So her father said, "Savitri, do not wait for someone to choose you. Choose for yourself a husband who will be your equal."

So Savitri searched for a man she could love and trust and presently found a prince named Satyavan who lived in a mighty forest. Satyavan was a young man with many great qualities such as intelligence, honor, integrity, courage, and compassion. However, for all his wonderful qualities, it was fated that Satyavan had only one more year to live.

The king said to Savitri, "Surely you can find another suitor whom you can grow old with?" For he did not want to see his daughter widowed and grieving in such a short time. But Savitri's mind was made up. She answered, "A thing is first thought of in the heart, then it is spoken of, and then it is done."

Seeing that her heart was intent on Satyavan whatever the consequences, the king blessed their union and the wedding was set.

Savitri married Satyavan and for one year they lived happily in his forest home until the day arrived that his death was fated. On that day, Savitri went to work with her husband in the woods and watched as he chopped one tree after the other. As the day wore on, Satyavan grew sick and faint and came to his wife saying his head was filled with darting pains.

Savitri sat on the ground, her heart wracked with sorrow at the thought of losing her beloved husband. But she smiled gently at him, for he did not know of his impending fate, and she said, "Come here, my love, lay your head in my lap and rest for a bit."

Satyavan closed his eyes and Savitri stroked his hair and wiped the sweat from his brow, singing softly to him. As she looked up, she saw a glowing, ruddy God before her. His eyes were dark and red, his face was monstrous, and in his hand he held a noose.

"I am Yama, Lord of Death," he announced. "I have come for Satyavan." And he drew the soul from Satyavan, leaving his body cold and lifeless. Then he started walking south with Satyavan's soul in his noose.

Savitri followed close behind.

Yama turned to her and said, "Go home, Savitri. It is not your time to go where we are headed. Go home and prepare your husband's funeral."

But Savitri would not go home.

She persisted after Yama until he offered her a boon. She asked that her father-in-law regain his health. This Yama agreed to, and then told her once more to go home. Once more she disagreed and continued to follow him, and he gave her another boon. Then another one, where she asked for one hundred sons for her father. This he agreed to, and then she asked for one hundred sons for her and Satyavan. This, too, Yama agreed to. Finally, Savitri beseeched the god, "You have promised me one hundred sons from the union between Satyavan and I, but you must give me my husband's life in order for this promise to come true."

Finally Yama agreed and gave back Satyavan, promising them both prosperity and long, well-lived lives.

And so it came to pass that Satyavan and Savitri bore many sons, and Savitri's father received his original request of one hundred sons through the wisdom of his daughter—his own gift from the goddess Sarasvati.

Ceremony for Sarasvati's Divine Guidance and Knowledge Before an Exam

Find a goddess statue to represent Sarasvati. You can use a tarot card or draw a picture of Sarasvati, or you can use an old Barbie doll if you like. Just dye her hair black and dress her in a white sari, which you can make from a piece of white cloth.

On your dressing table, make an altar for Sarasvati. Put a yellow cloth on the altar and place your Sarasvati figurine on it, facing east.

Decorate the altar with white and yellow candles and flowers. Marigolds especially are sacred to Sarasvati. Bring offerings to Sarasvati of berries or plums. She also loves Rice Krispies and yogurt.

Place your exam textbooks in front of Sarasvati and ask her to bless them. Whenever you are not using the textbook, leave it there on the altar for her to continue blessing.

On the morning of the exam, get up early and bathe, then dress in yellow or wear a yellow ribbon around your wrist in honor of the Goddess.

Say a prayer to Sarasvati:

Dear Sarasvati

Goddess of all knowledge

Fill me with your divine knowledge and wisdom

Bless my mind as I take this exam

May your confidence, grace, and knowledge flow through me

And inspire me as I take this exam

Light a candle and pass your hands over the top of the flame several times to warm them (not *in* the flame, mind you!). Pay special attention to the hand that you write with. Then touch your forehead with your hand and close your eyes. Imagine the power and knowledge of Sarasvati flooding though you, illuminating your mind with divine knowledge and understanding.

Go to your exam with confidence, knowing you have the blessing of Sarasvati with you. If you find yourself getting fear thoughts during the exam, close your eyes, visualize your altar, and say a quick prayer to Sarasvati for help.

Sacred Sexuality

In ancient India, the tantric arts were taught to young girls. Some girls devoted their lives to the practice of tantra. They were called *tantrikas*—priestesses or devotees of tantra. The movie *Kama Sutra* is about a young girl who became a tantrika. This is a beautiful movie that shows the skill involved in learning the arts of pleasure.

So what is tantra, and what were some of the tantric arts they learned?

Tantra is a philosophy and a way of life where sexual energy is used consciously as a creative energy. Tantrists know that whenever you make love with someone, something is always born of the union. This may be a physical child or it may be something quite different. Sometimes it is a feeling of complete love and bliss. Sometimes, if you sleep with someone who belittles you, it may be a feeling of unworthiness or loss of self-esteem. Every union bears fruit, whether good or bad. Tantrists use this knowledge to ensure every act of love between a man and a woman produces something of great beauty.

In tantra, sex is not separate from spirituality. Making love is a sacred act that is treated with honor and respect. The man and woman use makeup, clothing, and prayer to appear as a particular god and goddess before they make love, just as you do when you throw a glamour. The place where they will make love is always specially cleaned and purified, and they say special prayers to dedicate the area to the divine. They make the area as sacred as possible by burning incense, playing special music, and having fresh flowers—just like a temple space.

Then the couple says prayers to each other, honoring the God and Goddess in each other, before they make love. When they make love, they are making love as the God and Goddess. This experience is very magical. Not only does it bring you closer to your partner but it also brings you closer to the divine and to your spirit.

Tantra teaches that you can become a thing by identifying with it. So the more you focus your mind on a particular thing, the more like it you will become. If you focus on a person you hate, you will become filled with hate, or hate-full. If you focus on vengeance, you will become filled with bitterness. If you focus on a situation or person that gives you great pleasure, you will be filled with delight. When you focus on the Goddess, you become goddesslike.

Tantrikas would visualize in great detail the appearance and qualities of a goddess like Sarasvati or Shakti or Lakshmi. They would focus on a picture or statue of the Goddess, or see her clearly in their imagination. Their purpose was to focus with such devotion on the Goddess that they attained union with her. In order to practice tantra, a priestess must prepare her mind and body.

There were sixty-four skills that a priestess had to learn. Sarasvati is the patron goddess of the sixty-four arts of tantra, which include music, flower arranging, ceremonies, magic, dancing, singing, the art of conversation, and, most importantly, the art of love.

Goddess Workout

Today pay attention to people's countenances that you see around you. What do you think they spend most of their time thinking about? From the expressions on their faces, what qualities do you think they identify with most strongly?

179

Tantra Principles

The following are a few principles you can follow if you want to awaken your sexuality in a spiritual way. These exercises will kindle your sensuality.

Practice Loving Yourself

Fall in love with yourself! How do you do that? By treating yourself the way you would someone who you have a major crush on. Stop comparing yourself to other girls. Stop telling yourself horror stories about yourself or your life. Stop being mean to yourself in thoughts, words, or actions. Start building yourself up in your imagination. Tell yourself you can do anything with the power of the Goddess. Buy yourself flowers, take yourself out on a date, write yourself love letters.

Self-love is the most important step in tantra. When you don't love yourself, you may look outside yourself for someone or something to fill you up instead. You may seek validation from a boyfriend. This promotes insecurity, jealousy, fear of abandonment, and a tendency to cling. You may make your boyfriend's opinion of you more important than your own.

When you truly love yourself, you know that others are not your source. You feel happy with yourself, comfortable with your body, and accepting of where you are in your life. In other words, you like yourself. What you think of yourself is more important than whatever anybody else thinks of you.

Awaken Your Senses

Do things that bring pleasure to your senses. This will open the energy centers in your body and heighten your ability to receive and give pleasure. Sensuality is the doorway to sexual pleasure. By tuning into your senses, you fine-tune your ability to observe another's sensory reactions. Much of tantra's teachings involve feeding the senses. Sex is a sensual act. Tantrikas are skilled in using all their senses to arouse their partner. They know how to bring delight to a partner's senses, too.

....
Goddess Workout

To enhance your sight:

- Go to an art gallery
- Gaze at the sky
- Look in the mirror under dim lighting and imagine your face as the face of the Goddess

To enhance your hearing:

- Listen to silence
- Listen to nature
- Listen to your boyfriend's heartbeat
- Listen to the voice of spirit

To enhance your taste:

- Eat peeled grapes
- Eat ethnic food you have never tried before
- Eat melon dipped in honey
- Taste your boyfriend's skin

To enhance your touch:

- Massage body cream into your skin—notice the way your skin feels before and after
- Wear silky clothes
- Moonbathe naked
- Have a hot bubble bath

To enhance your smell:

- Wear your favorite perfume
- Wear your mom's favorite perfume
- Wear your grandmother's favorite perfume
- Walk around a restaurant and inhale all the different smells
- Go to the Body Shop and smell seven different essential oils

Cultivate Beauty

Add beauty into your life wherever you can. Have a beauty treat and do something special for yourself, like paint your toenails or give yourself a facial. Go to a drugstore and play with makeup or find some pretty ribbons and put your hair up. Buy some flowers for your bedroom. Turn your bedroom into a goddess temple. Put pictures of the Goddess up on the walls. Make an altar on your dressing table, and play soothing music and light candles. Create an act of beauty every day, like saying a kind word to someone or smiling at a stranger. Remember, the more beauty you put out into the world, the more will come back to you.

Choose a Boyfriend Worthy of You

Like Savitri, you must choose a boyfriend who is equal to you. Look for qualities that are sacred to you, like someone who is kind, compassionate, and respectful. What are the qualities that are important to you in a boyfriend? Do not go out with anyone who would belittle you or make you feel bad about yourself in any way.

Treat Your Body as a Sacred Temple

In tantra, your body is a sacred temple. Treat your body as you would any sacred temple. Be conscious of the substances you put into it. Eat healthy foods and do not abuse your body with cigarettes or alcohol. Exercise regularly, and bathe and groom yourself as a goddess. Do not let anybody be intimate with you who is not worthy of you. Your body is your holy temple and is sacred. Allow only those who would perform an act of devotion to you to be close to you—those who would worship you as the goddess you are. You are the priestess of your body temple and it is your responsibility to take good care of it, just as the ancient priestesses took good care of the goddess temples.

Chanting

Chanting can open all of the energy centers in your body. In a crisis, you can use chanting to help you clear your heart and mind. Chanting has a healing effect on the body and the mind, and can soothe a broken heart or calm an angry mind. Chanting can bring you closer to the Goddess and fill your heart with divine love and compassion. Chanting can also open you up to divine inspiration and is a wonderful technique to try when you are feeling blocked creatively. If you need to write a paper on creative writing or do a project for art or music class, try chanting for ten minutes first.

My favorite chant is one I learned in my first yoga class many years ago. It goes like this:

Om Namo

Guru Dev Namo

You can also practice chanting "Om" by itself. This is one of the most powerful chants in the universe. "Ma" is another chant you can repeat to invoke the presence of the Goddess.

Another chant I like is:

We all come from the Goddess

And to her we must return

Like a drop of rain

Flowing to the ocean

You can buy this chant and many others on CDs by Robert Gass (this chant is on *From the Goddess* [Boulder: Spring Hill, 1994]).

Practice chanting whenever you find yourself obsessing about something or someone, or when you are feeling down or upset.

"Embody the Goddess" Meditation

Lie down on your bed and feel your body sink into the mattress. Take nine deep breaths. With each breath, feel your body sink farther and farther into the mattress. Feel your whole body relax. You might like to have some soothing music playing while you do this. Now imagine that Sarasvati appears on the ceiling above you. You see her glowing with golden sparkles emanating from her body. She is dressed in her beautiful white goddess gown, with jewels and pearls decorating her body. She is smiling with kindness and love at you. She moves closer to you until she is right above your face.

You tell her any problems you might be having. You ask for her healing in any part of your body that feels stressed out. You pray for healing in any area of your school life that needs help.

If you are having any boyfriend problems, talk to her about these, too. Sarasvati was devoted to Brahma and will act as a "relationship guidance counselor" to you. She can also help you with any problems you might have concerning your sexuality.

Now feel the goddess move close to you until she merges completely with your body. Imagine your body becoming as brilliant as a million moons, just like Sarasvati's. Keep praying for divine help and thank Sarasvati for healing you. Visualize your heart, your body, and your mind as completely whole and healed. See your entire body made new by the divine power of the Goddess. If your heart was aching for any reason, see it made new by the power of Sarasvati.

Goddess Gazing

An ancient practice in India was to gaze upon the image of a goddess, looking into her eyes until you felt yourself embodying the energy of that goddess. Find a picture of a goddess that you like. You can use a picture of any woman that you like. If you have some tarot cards, you might like to use one of the cards with a picture of a goddess that appeals to you.

Take a shower and put your makeup on. In India, makeup has magical properties. When women put on their makeup for sacred ceremony, they are literally putting on the face of the Goddess. Kohl was used by both men and women in the East. Traditional kohl was prepared so it would clean and protect the eyes and feel cooling when applied. It darkens the rims so the eye appears erotically enticing. Eyes are sacred because they create a dramatic first impression. The first time you look into someone's eyes, you gain an impression of the energy of that person; whether their eyes are smiling or glaring tells you a lot about the person's inner character.

185

Once I met this girl whose demeanor was very sweet—she looked angelic with her tall, slender body and long, blonde hair. She always had a gentle smile on her lips and a quiet, soft-spoken voice. But when you looked in her eyes, there was such an intense depth of hate there it could almost knock you backwards. Quite literally, I would step back to distance myself from her energy.

So apply your makeup and then sit in a dimly lit room with your picture of the Goddess before you. Gaze at it steadily, without blinking, until your eyes start to water. Don't think about anything. Just keep your eyes focused on the picture. Feel yourself taking on the energy of the Goddess. Ask the Goddess if she has any messages for you at this time.

This is a great exercise for opening up your spiritual sight.

Sarasvati's Glamour

- ◆ White clothes—especially a long, white, sheer skirt or sarong

- ◆ Wear sandalwood perfume

- ◆ Shimmering white eye shadow

- ◆ A lotus blossom in your hair

- ◆ Mehndi decorations on your wrists

- ◆ A bindi on your forehead

- ◆ Stick-on stars by your eyes

Makeup

Apply a tinted moisturizer instead of a foundation, and dust your skin with a pearly powder, like Revlon's "Skinlights." Line your eyes with black eyeliner all the way around your eyes. If you can find a picture of an Indian goddess, use this to guide you. You want the eyeliner to be heavy on your upper eyelid and to extend outwards at the outside corner in a slight *V* toward the outer edge of your eyebrows. Then smudge slightly with your little finger.

186

Dust a pearly white eye shadow over your eyelids. Use black mascara to make your eyes look large and luminous. Use a pale pink blush on your cheeks and a pale pink lipstick on your lips.

Decorate around your eyes with tiny sparkly body gems that you can buy from the drugstore. Little hearts or stars are perfect. In between your eyebrows, stick a bindi. You can add a dab of glitter to the inside corner of each eyelid, too.

If you want to go for full priestess mode, you can drape a sheer white veil over your head.

Clothing

Do this ceremony in the evening. Run a bath. Put ten to fifteen drops of sandalwood or orange blossom essence into the water. Soak in the water and imagine you are floating on a lotus flower like Sarasvati. Allow the water to purify your body.

Pray:

Goddess, you can make all things new

Make my mind new

Make my heart new

Make my life new

When you are ready, get out of the bath and dress as Sarasvati. Put on white clothes, a sari, or a white nightgown. Wear pearls or sparkly jewels.

Ceremony

Now you are ready to invoke Sarasvati. Say a prayer to her:

Sarasvati

Goddess of wisdom, devotion, and sensuality

May your love pulse through my veins

May your beauty radiate from me

Give me the wisdom of my actions

Awaken in me my sacred sensuality

Lead me to those who would be devoted to me

Show me the power of my sexuality

May I guard it and use it wisely

Now go outside and meditate under the moon. Feel the energy of the moon fill your body. Dance under the moonlight—try belly dancing. Feel all your senses come alive. Plan a romantic evening for you and your honey, and the next time you kiss him, imagine yourself as Sarasvati.

Other Suggestions

- Drink milk sweetened with a little honey.

- Play Indian sitar music in honor of Sarasvati.

- Light a white candle.

Sarasvati's Tasks for You

- Practice observing people's eyes. Look deep into their eyes when they are talking to you. Notice what kinds of messages you are getting. Are they consistent with the words that are coming from the person's mouth?

- Make it your intention to do well in one of your classes that you have been finding difficult. Ask Sarasvati for her advice and take three actions to improve your performance. You could talk to your teacher and ask for help. Get an extra book out of the library, or ask a friend who excels in that subject to help you a couple of times a week.

- Go out into the world as Sarasvati one day this week. How does it feel to be the goddess of schoolwork and music?

- Find some music that you really enjoy and play it in honor of Sarasvati.

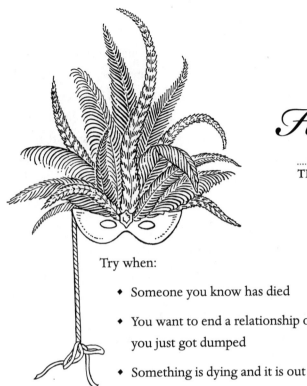

Huesuda

Try when:

- Someone you know has died

- You want to end a relationship or
  you just got dumped

- Something is dying and it is out
  of your control

- You need to banish something

Huesuda (pronounced *who-soo-da*) is the goddess who presides over death. According to my friend Elena, "We call her the Huesuda, which means 'The Bony One.' She is like the Reaper; she comes for us to take us to the other side. She is not considered a goddess, but Death itself."

Little figurines of Huesuda can be found around the time of the Mexican Day of the Dead on November 2. She is portrayed as a skeleton with black around her eyes and on her lips. She wears a long black gown and a black lacy veil over her head.

Huesuda is the goddess to go to when you wish to contact a family member who has already passed over. She can take messages from you to the other side. She is the goddess to go to when you just got dumped and feel like hell, or when you want to end a relationship. Huesuda appreciates the value of death and knows that for everything there is a season, a time to die, and a time to be reborn. She will help you understand death so you can let go of any fears you have concerning it.

She is also the goddess to go to when you want to end or transform something. If you have a habit or a friendship, a love relationship or a mistake that you or someone else made against you which hurt you, La Huesuda is the goddess to go to for help with banishing these things.

Huesuda's Story

As far as I know there is no special legend surrounding Huesuda. She is the goddess who brings candy to children on the Day of the Dead and who can take your prayers to God for the loved ones who have passed over. Although she looks like a scary figure—a skeleton wrapped in a black cloak with a bent-over frame—she is not frightening at all. She is more like a kindly old grandmother who comes to visit on the Day of the Dead.

The Day of the Dead (El Dia de Los Muertos)

The Day of the Dead is a Mexican holiday to celebrate the dead and to celebrate the continuity of life. The Day of the Dead is an ancient festival that goes back to Aztec times, way before Mexico became Christian. It is a time when Mexican families remember their ancestors and visit them at graveyards.

Originally, during Aztec times, the Day of the Dead was celebrated at the end of July or the beginning of August during the Aztec month of Miccailhuitontli, and was sacred to the goddess Mictecacihuatl, Lady of the Dead. However, after the Spanish conquest, the Catholic priests moved the festival to the beginning of November to coincide with the Christian holiday of All Saints' Day. This was an attempt to transform a Pagan event into a Christian one. Today the Day of the Dead is still celebrated in Mexico on November 2 with much gusto.

Families go to the cemeteries to visit their dead relatives. Everybody gets dressed up in his or her best clothes. This is a time of much festivity and celebration—not a time for grieving. When the family arrives at the graveyard, they tidy up their relatives' graves and decorate them with flowers and special mementos they have brought for their loved ones. They talk with friends who are visiting their loved ones' graves—the whole community joins in. They spread out a picnic by their relatives' graves and tell stories about the departed ones. The food quite often resembles a sumptuous feast. Families bring their loved ones' favorite foods. They make meat dishes in spicy sauces, cookies, chocolate, candies, and special breads made from an egg batter and shaped into bones, skulls, and animals. Marigolds and chrysanthemums are flowers that are sacred to the Day of the Dead, and families adorn the graves with a profusion of these brightly colored flowers.

People lay offerings of cigarettes, religious amulets, alcohol, and food on the graves, too, so the whole day resembles a large graveside party, where people join together, feast, tell stories of their loved ones, talk to their loved ones, and enjoy each other's company.

A special bread called *pan de muerto* is also prepared, and a plastic skeleton is cooked inside the bread. Finding the skeleton when eating the bread is a sign of good luck.

Goddess Workout

Make a loaf of pan de muerto, the "bread of death."

1½ cups flour

½ cup sugar

1 teaspoon salt

1 tablespoon anise seed

2 packets dry yeast

½ cup milk

½ cup water

½ cup butter

4 eggs

3–4½ cups flour

1. Mix all dry ingredients together except the 3–4½ cups of flour.
2. In a small pan, heat the milk, the water, and the butter. Add the liquid mixture to the dry mixture. Beat well. Mix in the eggs and 1½ cups of flour. Beat well some more.
3. Add the rest of the flour a little at a time until you have a dough mixture.
4. Knead the mixture on a floured board for 10 minutes.
5. Put the dough in a greased bowl and allow it to rise until it has doubled in size. This will take about an hour and a half.
6. Punch the dough down and reshape it, adding some bone shapes on top to decorate it. You could also shape it into an animal shape or an angel shape. If you like, now is the time to put a tiny plastic skeleton inside.
7. Let it rise another hour.
8. Bake at 350 degrees F (175 degrees C) for about 40 minutes.
9. After baking, sprinkle it with confectioners' sugar and colored sugar.

Little children and babies who have died are often remembered on November 1 as *angelitos* (little angels) and the adults are remembered on November 2. Before the Day of the Dead takes place, shops are filled with special items for the celebration. There are skeletons, brightly colored paper cutouts called *papel picado*, wreathes and crosses, candles, flowers, and edible treats in the shapes of skulls, coffins, angels, and other deathlike symbols. There are also little breads made in the shape of humans, which are called *animas* (souls) to represent the soul of the departed one.

At home, families make an altar for their relatives and decorate it with their purchases. They place papel picado, skeletons, flowers, candles, photos of their dead relatives, candy skulls inscribed with the relatives' names, and some of their favorite foods on the altar. The food often includes rice, beans, meat, atole (a corn gruel), beer or tequila, and chocolate, as well as any kinds of candy bars and soda that the deceased enjoyed. The feast is made as enticing as possible because the families expect a visit from the spirits of their dead relatives. They want to make the meal nourishing to provide adequate sustenance for the spirit's journey from the otherworld to this world, and back again!

A washbasin and freshly laundered towels are kept near at hand for the soul to freshen up before eating, too. Offerings of cigarettes are left out for relatives who smoked while they were alive, and there are many candles and some copal incense lit to light the way for the souls to find their way home. Relatives sprinkle marigold petals from a door to the altar to make a sacred pathway for the spirit to follow.

Goddess Workout

Make an altar on a dressing table for someone you loved who has died. Place fresh flowers, a photo of them, and some of their favorite foods on the altar, and call their soul to come visit you.

I did this once several years after my mother died. I cleared my kitchen table, where I set up the altar. I placed a photo of her and some of her special things on the table—a lipstick, her perfume, some jewelry, and a china plate she had painted for me. Then I made a salmon and sweet corn sandwich for her (her favorite), a piece of chocolate cake, and a cup of tea. I invited her to come join me. She did, and I got the distinct impression that she was cross with me for setting the altar up in the kitchen, which was quite drafty, as she would have preferred to be in a warmer room!

Contacting Loved Ones Who Have Died

How They Can Help You

When people die, they often have more energy to help you than when they were alive because they don't have all the day-to-day concerns of their own lives. People who love you enjoy helping you once they have passed over. They can help you with things that they were good at that you might want help in. For example, if your grandfather was a lawyer and you need some help with a legal matter, you can ask your grandfather to intervene and give you some support and help. If you had a relative who quit an addiction and you are trying to quit the same addiction, you can ask for help with this.

If you had a relative who was talented in a particular area that you would like to study, ask them for help, too. Like if you had a relative who was a writer and you need to write a paper, ask him or her for help, or if you are having car trouble and you had a relative who was a mechanic, ask him or her to lead you to the perfect garage to fix your car. We have so much help available to us from the spirit realms, it is crazy for us *not* to ask them for help!

How to Contact Them

To ask for help, all you need to do is say a prayer and have an offering ready for them. An offering can be anything they liked while they were alive—a favorite chocolate, a cigarette, a cookie, a flower, or a candle. Then just say a prayer:

Dear _____

Please come help me

I need help with . . .

You can also write letters to your loved one. Just put on some relaxing music and write a letter to your dead relative. I have found late at night or very early in the morning are the best times to do this. Then ask them questions and write down what you hear them saying. You can heal a relationship that was fractious while the person was alive in this way, too.

My mother died suddenly and we had a very difficult relationship the last few years of her life. Through the process of meditating and writing to her, and writing her answers, we have healed a lot in our relationship. Remember, when people die their soul still lives, so you can still have a relationship with them even though they are not physically present. You can ask them to send you a sign that they are

194

still around. Don't worry that you might be keeping them from being somewhere else in another dimension. Spirit beings can be in many places at the same time, as they are not bound to the same time and space limitations that we are. Your dead relative can be with you and your siblings all at once, even if you live miles apart.

Tracing Your Ancestry

Who are you and who do you come from? Who were the women in your lineage and what traits still run in your DNA? You have at your disposal an unlimited supply of power. The power of your ancestors flows through your veins via your DNA. What is your spiritual lineage? What is your physical lineage? All native traditions have a wide variety of skills and power—their own medicine, if you like. What are the skills your ancestry was renowned for? Call on the power of your ancestors to come to you now.

Honoring Endings

In our culture we are not really taught how to celebrate death. Death is supposed to be a time of great sorrow—a big ending followed by a drawn-out grieving process. However, suppose you knew that your loved one was going on to a better place and a happier life, like if someone you loved was going on a trip around the world to see all the things they had always wanted to see. Would you be sad for them? I doubt it. You would miss them, sure. But you would be happy and maybe a touch envious that they were going somewhere better. What if this was the case when people died? Many cultures believe that the afterlife is a better place than the mundane world.

What about if you go through the ending of something painful, like the breakup of a relationship, or you lose a job? What if you knew without a doubt that there was something better for you right around the corner? Would you still want to hold onto all your grief and agony about losing the old? There is a season to everything. When something dies, something else will be reborn. Even in the seeming bleakness of winter, new growth is stirring within the earth, waiting to manifest in the spring. And so it is in our lives. At every ending, every death, in those seemingly bleak, drought-filled periods of time, new shoots are busily preparing underground to be birthed again into something better, something more wondrous, for your life.

In my experience, nothing is ever taken without something better being given in return.

It is safe to trust the process of life

There is great wisdom in life

To every ending there is a new beginning

To every winter a spring

To every darkness a dawn

How to Celebrate an Ending

The next time something in your life doesn't work out and you face an ending, instead of wallowing in it, try something different. Spend a week dressed as Huesuda, wearing black every day to signal your period of mourning. Then, on the seventh day, have a party to celebrate your life and the new things that are coming. Clean up your room; get rid of all the clutter in a symbolic gesture of getting rid of the old to make room for the new. Wash your hair. Wear your brightest, most fabulous clothes. Buy or make cupcakes and decorate them with brightly colored sprinkles. Invite some friends over and celebrate "the best is yet to come." Celebrate the new boyfriend who is on his way, the new job that will soon be here, the new whatever it is that you wish to manifest in your life. Whenever a fear thought comes to mind, like "I'm never going to find someone else, another job, whatever . . ." quickly banish it and say out loud: "My new boyfriend is on his way," "My new job is waiting for me," or whatever it is you do want, and: "Endless opportunities and possibilities are opening up to me right now!"

....

Goddess Workout

What are your beliefs about immortality and the afterlife? Where do you think people go when they die? What do you think it will be like—how will it be different from your experience here on Earth?

I have read lots of interesting books on the afterlife. In the Celtic worldview, they believe that we go to the Summerland when we die. This is a magical, mystical place where there is lots of eating and drinking and partying with gods and goddesses.

In a book by Sylvia Browne, *Life on the Other Side*, Sylvia says when we die we move into the spirit world. We still appear in human form, but we look about thirty and there are all sorts of fun things to do in the spirit world. You can go to fashion shows, parties, study, read, and write. You can manifest whatever you want instantaneously, so you can change your appearance, get a new home, a new dress, or a new boyfriend all with the blink of an eye. This sounds like a great deal of fun to me.

What were you told about death as you were growing up? What would you *like* to believe about death now?

Endings and Banishing

Sometimes you may need a little help in moving the ending process of something along. In this case a banishing can be useful.

There are two very important components to learn in the practice of magic. One is the ability to manifest and the other is the ability to banish. What is banishing? It means to magically end something, to cast away the unwanted circumstance or person from your life and to undo any negative effects caused by it. When you banish in the name of magic, you are driving something out of your life by the power of the Goddess.

The dark moon is a great time for banishing and, because she presides over death, Huesuda is a great goddess to ask for help with banishing.

What Kinds of Things Can You Banish?

You can banish anything you no longer want in your life. These include but are not limited to:

- A friendship that is ending

- An addictive behavior

- A relationship where you don't want to go out with the person anymore

- A bad habit you may have

- Heartache and pain from a situation where others hurt you

- A quality in yourself that you want to change—like being impatient

How Do You Banish?

Well, there are many techniques for banishing, and they depend a lot on the situation. If it is a friendship or a relationship that you don't want to be in anymore, say a prayer to the Goddess:

Dear Goddess

The feelings of my heart have changed

I no longer want to be friends with _____

Please help me to end this in a way that is loving and honest

Help me to stay true to myself and not commit to anything

Out of a desire to please others at my own expense

I ask that you lead me toward the people who would best serve me at this time

And lead my friend/boyfriend to the people who would best serve their needs at this time

Please surround my friend with your loving comfort

May we both accept this change in a positive, transformative way for the good of all

And so it is

Then light a candle on the dark moon, or the full moon—whichever comes first—and say your prayer. Close your eyes and see your friend surrounded by the love of the Goddess and being gently guided toward people and situations that would best benefit her or him. You might like to write a letter to this person, thanking them for all the good things they brought into your life. Once when a friend decided to end a friendship with me, she wrote and told me she couldn't be friends with me anymore. So I wrote her a letter and thanked her for all the kind things she had done for me over the years. I felt sad at the ending of our friendship, but glad to be able to respect her boundaries and to express my heartfelt gratitude for what the friendship had meant to me.

Another time when a relationship I was in was breaking up, I was very sad. I got a beautiful crystal and held it in my hands and filled it with love from my heart. I imagined all the good things in our relationship, all the memories, happy and sad, and sent it to my ex. That way I was no longer holding all those memories in my heart, and I was free. You could put all the memories into a special stone and then bury it if you don't feel comfortable giving it to the other person.

A Spell to Banish a Heartache or a Bad Habit

What if the spell you need is for yourself? Let's say you have a bad habit or some pain and hurt that you have been carrying in your heart as a result of something that someone else's actions have caused. Well, the process is still the same.

First say a prayer:

Dearest Goddess

I don't know how to heal a broken heart

But you do

Goddess, you can heal anything and I am asking you to heal me now

Banish this pain to the realms of which it came

I ask that all the negative effects from this be undone

In all dimensions of time and space, right now

I ask that I see the gifts that have come from this

And that you strengthen my faith and comfort me

And so it is

Amen

Prayer for a Bad Habit

Dearest Goddess

I know that this habit no longer serves me

It does me more harm than good

I ask that you remove from me all thoughts, behaviors, and actions that trigger this habit

Remove also, dear Goddess, all effects of this habit from the past, present, and future

In all dimensions of time and space

I surrender my habit to you

I ask you to replace it with your divine love

And with divine guidance lead me toward habits that enrich my life

Send extra helpers right now to help me with this

Thank you, dear Goddess

And so it is

Amen

Then light a candle, say your prayer, close your eyes, and feel your body being filled with divine light and love. Whenever you start to feel the heartache arising or feel yourself wanting to indulge in the bad habit, repeat the prayer, close your eyes, and see the Goddess helping you right now.

A Spell to Banish a Person Who Is Causing You Harm

What if there is someone who is causing you trouble in your life? This may be someone who is mean-spirited, someone who envies you and always tries to steal from you—copies your ideas and passes them off as their own, tries to seduce your boyfriend, or puts you down in little and not-so-little ways. Or it could be someone who bullies you or is just generally unpleasant to be around. The less you have to do with this person, the better. Such a person is not a true friend. Often people who act this way are acting from jealousy or envy. They want something that you have.

Sometimes people deliberately set out to steal things from you. Another time this happened in my life with a girl who was jealous of me. She said, "Catherine always makes things work out for herself!" I think she didn't realize that *she* could make things work out for herself, too.

She began stealing things from me and started trying to create havoc in my life. She began flirting outrageously with my partner, talking about me behind my back, and just being a not-very-nice person. I knew in my heart that she was deeply unhappy with her own life, but even though I felt empathy for her I didn't want her doing her bad stuff around me. This was time for big magic! Talking with her wasn't working. She was not in a place where she was willing to reason anything. Her intentions were not good as far as I could see. So what to do?

Well, first of all, I handed the whole situation over to the Goddess. I made a point not to have anything more to do with her. I did a ceremony where I called upon the powers of my ancestors to protect me and my loved ones, and banished her from my life. Happily she is no longer a part of my life, in any way, shape, or form. I also prayed that any harmful effects from her actions toward me and my family would be undone in all directions of time and space.

The Spell

Do this on the full moon or the dark moon. Get a candle—black is good, or dark maroon or purple.

Say a prayer to Huesuda:

Dear Goddess

_____ is causing me a great deal of trouble

I no longer want her in my life

Please undo any effects of her actions toward me

In all dimensions of time and space right now

Through the power vested in me as a daughter of the Goddess

I banish _____ from my life from this day forward for the good of all

And so it is

In your imagination, see the person walking away from you without looking back—off to find a better future for herself somewhere else that doesn't concern you! Light the candle and let it burn down. When it has burned, bury the remnants in a graveyard somewhere or throw them into a living body of water. Flushing them down the toilet also works well. Make sure you wash your hands after handling the candle.

What if you have a situation regarding a family member whom you live with, and it is physically impossible to banish them completely from your life? You have to see them on a daily basis, at least till you leave home. Again, surrender the situation to the Goddess. Say a prayer:

Dear Goddess

I am really having great difficulty with my relationship with _____

I now place this relationship in your hands

I ask that any effects from all actions of mistakes they have made toward me

Be completely undone in all directions of time and space

I ask that any of my actions which may have upset _____

Be completely undone in all directions of time and space

I banish her ill will toward me for now and forever

In the power of the Goddess

I ask for divine protection and divine guidance to surround me now

And so it is

Sometimes there may be someone who is causing you difficulties who is not in your life by choice but because of circumstances. If this is the case, there are many ways you can take care of yourself when you are faced with this person. You can wear a tiny mirror around your neck so that any unkindness they direct at you is immediately reflected back to them. You can learn to not take their comments personally. You can learn how to empower yourself. You can learn to set boundaries by not spending time alone with them. You can learn to rely on the strength of the Goddess to get you through difficult moments.

Our worst enemies can sometimes be our greatest teachers. A great warrior becomes great by having worthy foes. So never let anyone get you down. Remember, you carry the power of the Goddess within you. Remind yourself by saying out loud:

I am a priestess of the Goddess

I carry the power of the Goddess within me

I can use magic to manifest what I want in my life

I can use magic to banish what I don't want in my life

I can call on help from the spirit world

My ancestors, the ancient priestesses, the angels, and my power animals

I am not alone in this

Indeed, I am loved and protected by the Great Goddess

Who is all-powerful, all-present, and all-knowing

And so it is

Huesuda's Glamour

- White skin (use theater or Halloween makeup)

- Lots of black eyeliner smudged around your eyes

- Absolutely no blush—the more deathlike you look, the better

- Dark purple lipstick

- Midnight blue eye shadow

- Black clothes—make sure you are dressed in black from head to toe

This is one of my most favorite glamours. When I was a teenager I loved to dress up all in black. I still do!

Makeup

Cleanse and moisturize your face. Put a pale foundation over your skin, then apply white Halloween makeup to give your face a ghostly glow.

Darken your eyebrows with black eye pencil. Around your eyelids apply lots of soft black kohl. Smudge it gently with your little finger. On your eyelids apply an eye shadow in a smoky color such as maroon, slate blue, purple, or gray. Take the color all the way up past the crease in your eyelid to your brow bone. Gently brush some eye shadow under your eyes, too. Now apply tons of black mascara— if you want to wear false eyelashes that is great, too, just follow the directions on the packet.

Color your lips in a deep burgundy, red, or purple. If you want to be ultra-dramatic, then try black lipstick. Wear nail polish in the same color as your lipstick ("Vamp" by Chanel is great).

Clothing

Wear anything black: long black lacy dresses, black pants, black silk shirts, black fishnet, black lace, black velvet. Other colors that also work to break the monotony of black are maroon, silver, tapestry, emerald green, ruby red, purple, or stark white.

For accessories, wear silver—and lots of it! Religious amulets, such as crosses or saints, black velvet chokers, and silver flowers or bats are also appropriate.

Hairstyle

Wash your hair (before you put your makeup on). Wrap it up in a towel while you are applying your makeup, then after your face is ready you can do your hair. Place a small amount of hair gel in the palm of your hands, rub them together, and then rub them through your hair. Blow-dry your hair, bending over at the waist and scrunching your hair with your free hand. When your hair is almost dry, flip your head up and apply a small amount of gel, scrunching it into your hair. Then lightly tease your hair with a comb and spray lots of stiff hairspray into your hair, especially at the roots.

Ceremony

Make an altar to celebrate the life of someone you loved who is no longer here. Share a meal of their favorite foods with them.

Invoke Huesuda to help you deal with any aspect of death. Pray:

Dear Huesuda

Please come to me now

Help me to know that even though

_____ is no longer here with me in body

They are still here with me in spirit

Huesuda's Tasks for You

- Have a gothic party to celebrate death. Decorate with red, black, and white candles. Invite your friends to come dressed as Goths and tell stories of people you have loved and their lives. Bring favorite foods of the people who have passed over.

- Is there someone you know who is close to death or elderly? Talk to them and see how they feel about dying. If you don't know anyone who is close to death, ask your family members how they feel about dying and what they would like their funeral to be like. Ask them what they would most like to be remembered for.

- Write your own will. You don't have to do this formally with a lawyer. In your goddess notebook, write down who you would like to get your stuff if you died suddenly. Also write down what you would like your funeral to be like—what kinds of food would you like there, what music? Where would you like to be buried or would you rather be cremated? What would you like to be remembered for? What would you like people to say about you at your funeral? Are you living your life in a way now that would cause people to speak about you as you wish, or are there some changes that you need to make. Ask the Goddess to help you make any changes.

- What if you only had one year left to live? How would you live it? We all have been lulled into a false sense of security to some extent, thinking that our lives will stretch out for many years. But we never know when the moment of death may come upon us. Tragic events, like the World Trade Center explosions, make us aware of our mortality. We can use events like that to motivate us toward making every day count. Life is a precious gift and we never know when it will be taken from us. Use your time here wisely.

- Celebrate death. Have your own private funeral to mark the ending of a relationship. Be Huesuda for a while, until you feel ready to move on again.

207

Celebrate your life
every day!

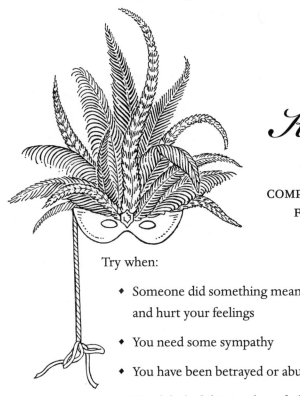

Kuan Yin

GODDESS OF
COMPASSION AND
FORGIVENESS

Try when:

◆ Someone did something mean to you
and hurt your feelings

◆ You need some sympathy

◆ You have been betrayed or abused

◆ You did a bad thing and you feel guilty

Kuan Yin (pronounced *qwan yin*) is the goddess of mercy and compassion from the Buddhist religion. She was originally from India and is today widely worshipped in China.

Kuan Yin helps couples that don't have any children to conceive, and heals the sick. She is the patron goddess of travelers and farmers and she protects souls in the underworld. She guides all those who are searching spiritually to enlightenment. She even made a vow not to leave this planet until all souls were enlightened!

Most Chinese deities are worshipped in temples but some, like Kuan Yin, are worshipped in people's homes. Little figurines of Kuan Yin are quite likely to be found on a dressing table with offerings left to her in the form of flowers and pennies.

Kuan Yin knows all about forgiveness and compassion. She will help you heal from wounds that are so deep and painful you can't even speak of them. Her father set fire to the nunnery where she lived in an attempt to murder her and still she was willing to have her hands cut off to save his life!

Her name means "she who hears the weeping world." When you weep, Kuan Yin will come to your aid and pour her loving compassion into your heart.

Kuan Yin's Story

Kuan Yin and the boys by the Yellow River

Once upon a time, a long, long time ago, there was a little village in old China that sat upon the banks of the Yellow River.

Early one summer's morn there appeared a mysterious young woman of extraordinary beauty. She was petite in stature, with large black almond-shaped eyes and delicate upward-arched eyebrows placed on an oval face with porcelain skin so pearly it appeared luminescent. Framing her face was her soft, wavy, long black hair. She moved as gracefully as the swaying of a lotus flower in a gentle breeze, and indeed the soft scent of the lotus blossom seemed to follow her wherever she was.

The young woman carried a basket in her hands woven from bamboo. This basket was lined with green willow leaves from the ancient weeping willow trees and was filled to overflowing with fish with golden scales gathered from the Yellow River.

All the villagers wondered where she came from, as the beautiful young woman sold her wares along the river. But no one knew who she was or from whence she came.

Each morning she appeared and as soon as her basket was empty she disappeared so quickly that the villagers wondered if she had been there at all or was just an apparition.

Now the young men of the village watched her with much interest, delighting in her beauty and graceful movements. One morning, unable to contain their curiosity any longer, they stopped her on the path and begged her to marry them.

But she answered in a lilting voice:

"O honorable young gentlemen, I do wish to marry; however, I cannot marry you all! If there is one among you who can recite the entire Sutra of the compassionate Kuan Yin by heart, then he shall be the one I will wed."

Now, none of the boys had ever heard of the Sutra of Kuan Yin, let alone memorized it. They were far more interested in sports and fishing than prayers and goddesses. But the next evening they met and egged each other on and by dawn, when the maiden appeared again, there were thirty of them who could recite the text by heart.

The young woman exclaimed, "Why, there are thirty of you and only one of me! Surely I cannot marry thirty of you. But if any one of you can explain the meaning of the Sutra, then he is the one I shall wed."

The next morning, ten hopeful young men were waiting to claim the maiden in marriage, for they understood the writings of the sacred text. But again the young woman said, "I cannot marry all ten of you, for I am only one woman. But if in three days any one of you has experienced the meaning of the Sutra, then I will gladly marry him."

On the third day there was one young boy waiting for her on the side of the riverbank. His name was Mero, from the house of Me.

The young girl's face lit up when she saw him. "Oh, Mero," she exclaimed, "I see in your heart that you have indeed felt the meaning of the blessed Sutra of Kuan Yin. I gladly accept you as my husband. Come to my house this evening and meet my parents. My home is by the river's bend." And with that, she was gone once more.

Mero was so excited; he went home and washed his hair and put on his finest clothes. All day he polished and primped himself in eager anticipation of the evening before him. As twilight fell, he walked to the river's bend, where he found a little cottage hidden among the reeds and rocks. There at the gate stood an old man and woman with their arms outstretched toward him.

"I am Mero, the son of the house of Me," he announced. "I have come to marry your daughter."

The old man smiled and said, "We have been waiting for you for a long, long time. You are very welcome here, young Mero."

And the little woman gently took him by the arm and guided him into the cottage to her daughter's room.

But the room was empty. From the open window he saw a stretch of sand leading down to the river and in the sand were the footprints of the young woman. Mero raced down to the water's edge where he found two golden sandals. Anxiously he looked down the river. He looked up the river. He looked over the river. All to no avail. There was no trace of the beautiful young woman. And as the sky darkened around him and night fell, he looked back to the cottage and saw that it had disappeared.

There he was, all alone, with only the rustling of the bamboo and the clapping of water against the rocks to keep him company. As Mero stood alone on the shores, listening to the beating of his heart, he closed his eyes in despair.

"Where are you, my beloved?" he called out with his mind. "Why have you forsaken me?"

And in a flash the young fisher girl appeared in his mind, as beautiful as ever. Transfixed, he watched as her features melted away, revealing the wise, compassionate face of Kuan Yin herself.

Suddenly he understood. The young fisher girl was none other than the goddess Kuan Yin herself. Kuan Yin whispered gently, "Mero, let your heart merge with mine. Open your heart to me."

And Mero felt his heart burst open and he felt the divine lovingkindness and compassion of Kuan Yin fill his soul. He had never felt love like this before. His heart was bursting with love and compassion and he knew he had received enlightenment from the Goddess.

Mero understood in that moment that their marriage was a spiritual union rather than a physical bond. He knew that Kuan Yin would continue to pour her love and compassion into his heart day after day and strengthen his connection to the divine realms. And in return he would radiate her love and compassion to those around him on the earthly plane until he crossed over to the other side and would dwell with Kuan Yin forever.

"You made a bridge of love," he called out to her in prayer, "that I might cross to the shore of Bodhi, and know enlightenment. Thank you, blessed bodhisattva, thank you." And Mero went home and carried the gifts of Kuan Yin within his heart forever.

Learning Kuan Yin's Loving Forgiveness

Forgiveness is one of the most powerful spiritual practices you can learn. I used to think I knew a lot about forgiveness, but one day I discovered that I really knew nothing about it. I would say I had forgiven someone for something they did that hurt me, but years later I would still be carrying around the hurt and pain and resentment whenever a memory of that incident came to my mind. When you have truly forgiven a situation that caused you pain, you no longer feel any emotional charge when you remember the situation. It is just like watching a mental movie that leaves you with no particular feeling—as if you are seeing an ad on TV about something you have no interest in.

Forgiveness sets you free. It does not mean you condone the behavior or the actions of the person who hurt you. It does not mean that you still have to be friends with that person if you no longer want to be. It does not even mean that you have to understand why the situation occurred or what motivated the person to act as they did. Perhaps you may never understand, and that is okay, too.

Forgiveness cuts the etheric cords that still bind you to the person and the situation through your pain, grief, and any other emotions. As long as you hold blame, resentment, hurt, or bitterness in your heart around the situation and the person, you are still attached to them. Your hurt does not hurt them—it hurts you. Your bitterness does not hurt them, it hurts you, and the same truth holds forth for any other emotion you feel toward the situation or person.

By holding on to pain and resentment, you are allowing your own personal power to leak away. Be willing to let go of grief and resentment and to open your heart to the healing power of self-love and forgiveness.

213

What to Forgive

Make sure you are clear inside yourself for what you are forgiving. Like I said, you can forgive someone else for causing you pain, but you do not need to condone the behavior or incident that led to your pain—you want to release your feelings surrounding your experience of it. Resentment, bitterness, blame, and hate are poisons that pollute the waters of your life. As you release the past, you purify your inner emotional river so that it may flow sparkly clear within you once more.

When to Forgive

You will know when it is the right time for you to forgive. Knowing when is the right time to forgive is important. If a situation has occurred recently that caused you a great deal of pain, you may not feel ready to forgive. If this is the case, be honest with yourself about it. You may be carrying a great deal of anger and hurt, and these feelings can be very important while you figure out how you want to deal with the situation.

Talk to Kuan Yin; explain your dilemma to her. Anger can be a wonderful tool for setting boundaries. When you are angry at someone because of the way they have treated you, you can figure out how you *do* want to be treated and start putting some boundaries in place to ensure you get treated accordingly. Your anger may tell you that you no longer want this person in your life, or it may show you that you need to communicate how you feel and what is important to you. It may show you what is unjust about the situation and lead you to a way of finding personal justice. Standing up for yourself and protecting what is yours are two important tasks for goddess girls to know how to do.

Goddess Workout

Have a conversation with Kuan Yin in your mind. Tell her what you are still angry about. Tell her what you are still in pain about. Tell her everything that is on your mind about the situation. Ask her to help you see the situation in another way so that you can become willing to release your hurt and let the healing waters of forgiveness pour over you. Ask her to hold you in her heart of compassion and to walk with you through your grief and soothe your turbulent emotions.

What Forgiveness Will Do for You

Forgiveness will set you free from the binds that tie you to whatever or whoever has hurt you. As long as you hold hatred, resentment, blame, or bitterness in your heart toward someone who has injured you in some way, you are binding yourself to that person on the invisible realms. Once you forgive, you cut those binds loose—you may feel a great weight lift off your shoulders, and the flow of life will once more flow through you. Your heart will no longer be blocked and will become an open channel once again through which you can open up to all love, all goodness, and all mercy.

How to Forgive

Let Kuan Yin and her angels tell you what you need to do in order to truly forgive another and be set free yourself.

Forgiveness is a very personal act of compassion. A while ago I was having a very difficult time forgiving someone who did something that hurt me deeply. I wandered around all day in my mind saying, "How dare she do that to me!" I struggled with my hurt, my grief, and my absolute anger at being treated that way. There was nothing I could do to change the situation and that really pissed me off. I wanted to hurt her back. I wanted to lash out and hurt other people involved in the situation. However, I knew because of the law of cause and effect that if I kept putting angry energy out into the world, that was what I would get back—and I didn't want that.

What I truly desired was to be free of the situation, to not have to carry it around with me anymore because it was making me feel lousy. What I really wanted was angelic amnesia to block out all the feelings of pain and upset associated with the event. I didn't want to keep thinking about it and, in effect, re-living it every time I thought of it. I just wanted it to be over and done with.

So I prayed to the Goddess and to my angels one night for help. "Show me what I need to do to forgive," I asked. I did a wonderful forgiveness meditation before I went to sleep and I felt at peace. All night long, I had the most horrific nightmares. I woke up at 2 A.M. in a cold sweat and berated the Goddess and my angels. "What was that all about?" I asked. "I thought you were going to help heal me, not bring more pain to my consciousness!" I drifted back to sleep and had the most incredible dream where I was dressed like an angel and I took flowers to the girl. I felt so good inside by doing that.

When I woke up, I knew what I needed to do. As if in a trance, I drove to the florist and bought a flower and then left it on the girl's doorstep. I experienced a great flood of relief and freedom. I felt cleansed inside. For the first time in weeks I felt truly free. It was over and done with. My feelings of anger no longer bound me to her. I did it for me—not because I expected anything from her in return. Forgiving the situation healed me. I still don't think what happened was fair (it wasn't—well, not according to me, anyway). She is not someone I want to be friends with anymore. But I can sever my ties with her through the act of forgiveness and thus allow myself to move forward in love and peace.

Remember, strength and healing come from your connection to the Goddess.

Goddess Workout

Write down the name of someone who has hurt you deeply. Light a blue candle and put some soft music on your stereo. Ask Kuan Yin and her priestess helpers to tell you what you need to do to forgive this person. Ask them to show you very specifically the steps you can take to be truly free of the etheric cords that bind you to him or her. Write down in your goddess journal what they say.

Coping with Revenge Thoughts:
The Law of Cause and Effect

Wanting to take revenge on someone who has made you feel deep anger or pain is pretty normal. Acting on those thoughts is not. There is a big difference between standing up for yourself and setting out to hurt someone else. Standing up for yourself and protecting your rights is using your goddess power wisely. Letting someone walk all over you is not using your goddess power. Setting out to hurt someone intentionally is BAD! When you sow seeds of bitterness and resentment, what are you going to get back? More of the same. Will intentionally hurting someone else make you feel better about yourself? Will it make you feel better about the situation?

I love the quote, "Resentment is like taking poison and expecting someone else to die."

Watch your words, too. When you say mean things about someone or wish something terrible would happen to them, you are, in effect, cursing them. You are hurling your anger and bitterness into the future.

When revenge thoughts seem overwhelming, write them out on your computer or a piece of paper. Write whatever you wish. Write fast until you have got all the mean things out that you want to get out. When you are done, delete the file or throw the piece of paper away. Say, "I no longer choose to carry these around with me." Repeat as many times as necessary. Hand the entire situation over to Kuan Yin and ask her to heal your heart.

Rest assured that what goes around, comes around. You don't need to worry about getting revenge. People trip themselves up eventually with their own intentions.

Forgiving the Unforgivable:
Turning Wounds Into Sacred Scars

What if the situation seems unforgivable? There are many incidents that in my eyes seem unforgivable—child abuse, rape, the Holocaust, violence to the elderly. Do you have to forgive these incidents? My view is nothing will make a wrong right, whether it is a big thing or a "little" thing. However, you also don't have to let the situation define who you are in a way that robs you of power.

All spiritual warriors carry battle scars. These are sacred scars that you can wear proudly. "I was defeated and I arose from the ashes" is a much better view than "I was defeated and now everything in my life will be affected adversely because of it."

Forgiveness means letting go of the absolute agony and despair and taking charge of your life again. Many people who have become powerful activists lobbying for human rights have done so because of their own experience in an "unforgivable" situation.

Forgiving does not mean understanding why something happened. You don't have to understand something in order to forgive it. Forgiveness sets you free to take right action instead of inappropriate action. Forgiveness washes you clean of powerlessness and despair.

Goddess Workout

Take a pen and paper and write down all the people who have ever hurt you. Write down the little hurts and the big hurts. Name teachers, friends, strangers—anyone who said something or did something that caused you to feel hurt. Write down what it was that hurt you. Go through your entire past and just write whatever comes to mind. You may find yourself remembering incidents that happened a long time ago. Whatever comes up, write it down on your piece of paper.

Pray to Kuan Yin. Have a conversation with her in your mind. Tell her all these things that have caused you to feel hurt, angry, resentful, or bitter. Ask her to cleanse your heart by pouring her healing water, her vase, which contains the dew of compassion, into your heart. Feel her compassion and understanding filling your heart and radiating through your entire body. Feel the sacred water purifying and cleansing every cell in your body. You might like to take a shower and visualize her pouring water over you.

Ask her to remove the effects of the incident that hurt you. Say, "I release all negative effects from the incident in every dimension of time and space now. I let go of any attachment that I have to pain, anger, hurt, resentment, blame, and bitterness surrounding this situation and persons now. I ask to see this situation in another light so I may feel peace. I send all the pain and hurt into your loving hands, Kuan Yin, and know that you are filling my heart with love in its place."

Steps to Forgiveness

You don't have to cower before anybody. Sometimes forgiveness is seen as an act of weakness. Actually it is an act of incredible power. This does not mean turning the other cheek and allowing someone to walk all over you again. If you believe and act as if you are weak, a victim, or helpless, then you disconnect yourself from the divine source of Goddess power. The Goddess is not weak or helpless, and she is certainly not powerless. Her power flows through your veins and you can use it at all times. Always remember: in any situation, you have a choice.

Sometimes people hurt others through their own ignorance, poverty, or confusion. Sometimes people don't intend to hurt you but you may be hurt as a result of a misunderstanding, your own expectations, or a mistake. Some people may genuinely wish you harm.

Protecting Yourself from Those Who Wish You Harm

Turn to the chapters on Queen Boadicea and Mahuika to learn how to do a lorica to protect you from harm. Just know that all the power, strength, and protection of the Goddess is available to you at all times. You have no need to fear anybody, even if they seem set on hurting you. Simply pray to the Goddess and surrender the situation into her hands. Invoke the power of the Goddess within you before you leave home in the mornings. Say, "I believe in the power of the Goddess. This divine power is far greater than any human power. I now allow the power of the Goddess to flow through me. I know I am divinely protected, divinely guided, and divinely loved at all times."

Staying Friends After a Betrayal

If a friend has hurt you deeply, how can you decide if you want to stay friends with her or not? Deciding to stay friends with someone is a very personal decision, one that may take some praying to figure it out. Listen to your intuition. What does it tell you? Your intuition will guide you as to whether it is right for you to stay friends or not. Pray to Kuan Yin; ask her whether it is in your best interests to stay friends. There have been friends I have continued to hang out with after being hurt by them and there have been those I have cut from my life. It really depends on the situation.

Once one of my friends betrayed me badly. I was very hurt at the time. However, I thought about it a lot. I really liked my friend, even though I didn't like what he had done. He was a good person who had been going through a hard time, and he had made some not-so-good choices. Over the years he had been a wonderful friend to me, so I decided I wanted to give him another chance. I realized bad judgment leads to experience, which leads to good judgment. Sometimes the biggest mistakes people make can be their greatest learning experiences. I know this has been the case for me—I have made my fair share of mistakes.

Another time, when a friend let me down badly, I decided not to continue the friendship. There had been a series of little letdowns, subtle putdowns in the form of snide remarks, and then bigger betrayals, such as making out with guys I liked in my apartment and copying stuff that I did to the point where I felt like I was going to suffocate. One day I simply decided I had had enough and that was that. I just didn't want to be friends with her anymore.

You will know inside whether to stay friends or not. It may take a little while to decide, but just know that you will know!

If you do decide to continue the friendship, it is important to clear the air and then give your friendship a fresh start. You can't hold on to all the anger, resentment, or blame and still have a good friendship. Those feelings will slowly poison the relationship. Plus, that is not really forgiving them. Forgiveness means not holding the situation against them anymore but putting it in the history archives, where it now belongs.

So if you do want to stay friends, be willing to talk about what happened. Clear the air—ask the Goddess to help, and then be willing to let go of your feelings about it. How do you do that?

Change the Way You View the Situation

You don't have to accept the unacceptable. However, your attitude and feelings around a situation will either energize you or rob you of your power and energy. If you constantly think of yourself as a victim and say things like "This was the worst experience I have ever had" or "I can't believe they would do something so mean to me," you are giving your power away. When you keep reliving the situation in your mind and playing it over and over again, like watching a video fifty thousand times, and with each replay you experience the same hurt, the same anguish, and the same sense of betrayal and resentment, you are continuing to give your power away to the situation.

You can choose to stay stuck in the woundedness of a situation, or you can choose to move forward.

The first step to moving forward is to stop replaying the mental movie. How do you do this? Every time a thought about it arises, or an image of the hurt, turn your mind to something else. In other words, press the "eject" button in your mental video player, then put a new video in. I have found memorizing a prayer to be very effective with this. Every time a picture comes to mind of a situation that caused me pain, I say a prayer or affirmation.

The prayer I like to say comes in part from Louise Hay's book *You Can Heal Your Life* (Carlsbad: Hay House, 1984). It goes: *In the infinity of life where I am, all is perfect, whole, and complete. I believe in a power far greater than myself. This power is available to me at all times. I now allow this power to flow through me. I know all love, all healing, all solutions, all possibilities; all new creations come from this power. I open my heart to the healing power of the goddess right now. All is well in my world. And so it is.* Actually that is not exactly the way the prayer goes, but that is my version of it. I keep saying the prayer over and over till there is no room in my mind for anything else.

With every situation it is always better to view the gifts gained than the wounds inflicted. This seems more challenging with situations where you have experienced a deep sense of pain; however, it is not impossible. Look for the gifts you have gotten. Sometimes you may have to dig deep to see them but they will be there. Gold is found in dirt, remember. Maybe you have learned a lot about what kinds of people you can trust and what kinds you can't. Maybe you have learned how resilient you are. Maybe you have learned empathy for other people who experience a similar situation. Maybe you have discovered who your true friends are.

....

Goddess Workout

Make a list of all the lessons you have learned from the situation. What are the nuggets of gold you have found?

1.

2.

3.

Reframing the Language You Use and the Way You Think

When you talk about the situation from this point forward, use language that empowers you rather than casts you as a victim. For example, instead of saying "That was the worst thing that ever happened to me," say "That was the greatest learning experience of my life" or "That was the most challenging experience of my life so far." Here are some more examples.

Life-defeating phrases:

- I was devastated.

- I will never get over this.

- I hate him.

- I'm sooooo hurt.

- It's not fair.

- They crushed me.

- He broke my heart and I will never love anyone again.

Life-empowering phrases:

- I have arisen victorious.

- I walked through it and I emerged stronger.

- I let go of any attachments to him, good or bad. I choose only good for myself. All other people and conditions now disappear from my experience and find their good someplace else.

- I am resilient.

- Life happens, I can cope with it.

- I take charge of my life and make it better for me.

- My heart cracked open and now I can experience deeper love and deeper empathy.

How to Forgive Yourself

What if you have done something that you feel bad about? Maybe your actions have hurt someone else, or you have violated your own principles or values. If so, consider some steps you can take to heal the situation.

While you can't go back into the past and change events, you can do a lot to heal the effects of past actions.

Think about the situation. Who was harmed by your actions? How were they harmed? What could you do now to put things right? Pray to Kuan Yin for guidance and help.

Perhaps an apology is in order. You could write a letter to the person involved, or go see him or her. Maybe you need to make monetary compensation or some other kind of compensation to clear the air.

If you feel nervous about contacting the person but would like to do it, then pray for courage. If it is inappropriate to contact the person, you can still take action to clear the effects.

....

Goddess Workout

Lie down and close your eyes. Visualize the incident as you remember it. See all the people who were involved, and those who were affected by your actions.

Ask Kuan Yin and your angels to come to you now. Ask that all effects of your mistake be undone now in all dimensions of time and space. Ask Kuan Yin to send her healing energy into the lives and hearts of all affected by your actions.

Tell Kuan Yin that you are truly sorry for your wrong actions, and that you are willing to take action to remedy the situation. Ask her for suggestions as to what you can do. Write down what she says.

Then close your eyes once more and ask her to heal your heart from any guilt or shame surrounding the situation. Ask that all effects from the incident be removed from your consciousness now, and that all that remains are the lessons learned.

Kuan Yin's Glamour

- Chinese embroidery of any kind

- Asian-inspired prints

- Silk pajamas

- Lotus flowers

- Pale blue jewels

- Chopsticks in your hair with your hair gently pulled back into an up-do

- Kuan Yin's makeup is luminous and hauntingly beautiful

- Glow-in-the-dark lipstick and nail polish

Makeup

Use a luminous foundation one shade lighter than what you normally wear. You want your skin to look kind of ethereal. Apply a silver glitter eye shadow over your entire eyelid. You can use a very pale blue cream eye shadow instead, if you like. Next apply a dark blue liquid eyeliner to your eyelid from the inner corner of your eyes extending all the way out past the corner of your outer eye with an up-ward stroke. Don't use any eyeliner underneath your eyes.

For blush, use a pale pink in a shade that suits you. For lipstick, try a glow-in-the-dark one or a pale silver or a glossy pink lipstick.

Clothing

Choose anything that has an Asian feel to it, like the suggestions above. An alter-native is to wear a long, flowing pale blue skirt with a shimmery blue tube top.

For jewelry, moonstones are sacred to Kuan Yin, as are any pale blue jewels. You could wear a choker with a flower on it, or a sparkly blue pair of earrings.

Hairstyle

Wear your hair loose and flowing like Kuan Yin, or pulled back into an up-do, as she is sometimes pictured. You can put lotus flowers in your hair, or chopsticks. If you can't find lotus flowers, use orchids, tiny baby's breath, or pale blue flowers. Stick-on hair gems in blue and clear are also a good choice.

Ceremony

On the night of a full moon, leave a vase or glass filled with water outside and ask Kuan Yin to charge the water with her dew of compassion.

Dress in your Kuan Yin clothing and makeup, and hold the vase in your hands by your heart. Pray:

Kuan Yin

Goddess of love, mercy, and compassion

I know that you can heal all hurt

No hurt is too big or too small for you to heal

I open my heart to your peace and compassion now

Fill my heart, O Goddess, with compassion and mercy

Fill my mind with peace and understanding

Help me to practice forgiveness to those who have wronged me

I ask you to weave a cloak of compassion and mercy around me

May my heart radiate your peace and compassion right now

I am illumined with the love of the Goddess

Guide me and protect me on this day

And so it is

Anoint your heart with the water from the vase. Keep the vase on your altar, and at the end of each day sprinkle some of the water over you to wash away any hurts that may have occurred during the day.

Kuan Yin's Tasks for You

- Dress as Kuan Yin one day this week. Go out into the world as the goddess of peace, mercy, and compassion. Write in your goddess journal about your experience.

- Choose one situation of betrayal that still causes you pain, and ask for help from Kuan Yin in dealing with it. Memorize a prayer that you like—you can use the one I use, if you wish. Whenever the situation comes to mind, repeat the prayer, fifty times if necessary, until you feel peace of mind.

- Once you have forgiven someone, refuse to bring the situation up again even if you are having a fight with them. If the situation comes up in your memory, deliberately choose to think about something else or go do something else to change your focus.

- Forgive yourself for something you have done that went against your values. Make amends where necessary.

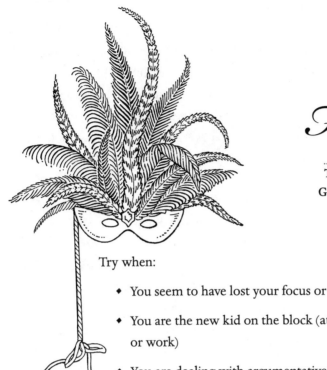

Freya

THE AIR
GODDESS

Try when:

- ♦ You seem to have lost your focus or direction

- ♦ You are the new kid on the block (at school or work)

- ♦ You are dealing with argumentative people

- ♦ You want new ideas, inspiration, and assistance with decision making

Freya (pronounced *fray-a*), the goddess of air, is the goddess of the east who rules the realm of the intellect. She carries the sword of illumination. The sharp blade of her sword is symbolic of her intellectual ability to cut through ignorance and confusion. The air goddess brings mental healing, inspiration, and clarity. She encourages you to use your awareness wisely. Clear thinking is an important quality for any goddess girl.

The Air Goddess is in charge of new beginnings and spring-cleaning. She is the goddess of spring, dawn, and the new moon. Her cleansing winds can sweep through you to blow away outworn attitudes, rigid ideals, and old values and beliefs. She will help you to let go of ways of thinking and blocked emotions that keep you stuck.

The Air Goddess rules clarity and illumination. When you ask her, she will help you to see yourself and those around you clearly. She will help you to discriminate in the decisions you make and the people you choose to bring into your life. She will throw light on false perceptions so you may see your life in focus. She bestows the gift of creative energy on you so you are filled with inspiration and new ideas. Her swordlike intellect provides you with the focus and determination to carry these ideas out.

The Air Goddess is a mentally strong and competent woman. She enjoys stimulating conversation and does not suffer fools easily. She is extremely intelligent and contains her power so she can use it effectively in a moment's notice. She will counsel you to use your mental power wisely and teach you how to deal with argumentative people and mental ailments.

There are stories of air goddesses in many different cultures. Freya is an air goddess from Norse mythology. She is also the goddess of rain and fertility, as the rain caused vegetation to grow. Freya wore a beautiful cloak that looked like a cloud, which acted as a barometer of her moods. When she was happy the cloud cloak would lighten in color, and when she was sad it would darken like a raincloud. When she was angry the cloud cloak became a thunderous storm cloud.

Freya's Story

The love story of Freya and Odin

Once upon a time, a long, long time ago, there was a beautiful goddess named Freya. She was the most beautiful and best-loved goddess of all the goddesses in Norse land. Freya had golden hair and snow-white skin. Her eyes were as blue as sapphires and sparkled like diamonds. She was tall, with a sweep of golden hair that reflected the sun like sparks of crystal as she shimmied her head from side to side.

Now Freya was married to Odin, the god of passion and intoxication. He was also the god of pleasure and love. Never had the villagers seen a more radiant couple. So in love with each other were they that everywhere they went together, all of nature blossomed and bloomed. Birds would come out to sing, flowers would dance, and trees would bear fruit just as Freya and Odin walked by. Their love was intoxicating and whoever came into their midst was affected by it. When they were apart, winter fell, and Freya's heart froze with ice. The lands would become barren, no birds would sing, and the trees would shed their leaves and wait for the warmth of love to feed them once more.

Odin loved Freya with all his heart, and most of the time he lived happily with her in their home with their two daughters. But Odin was also an adventurer. He loved to go off and see the world. Staying home with his wife and two daughters was difficult for him. He felt antsy and yearned to travel. His was a restless heart.

So one day Odin packed up a small bag with a few of his belongings and left his wife to go seek some new adventures. Freya was heartbroken. Her grief was inconsolable. Without Odin she was like the sky with no sun, the stars with no sky, and the forest with no trees. For many days and many nights, Freya sat upon the rocks outside her home by the ocean and wept ceaselessly. As her tears fell upon the rocks, they softened into sand. As her tears fell into the sea, they at once became precious amber. Freya cried and cried, but to no avail. Odin did not appear.

Finally, one morning Freya awoke after another restless night dreaming of her beloved Odin. Her heart was as heavy as lead, her head pounded from anguished grief, and her eyes were bleary from the thousands of tears she had shed.

"Enough!" she said. "If Odin will not come home, then I must go off in search of him." And with that she set off with her children to find her husband, for her life was barren without him by her side. She longed to hold him in her arms and in her heart once more. At each village she came upon, Freya would ask, "Have you seen my husband, the great god Odin?" But at each village she would receive the same answer. "No, my lady, he has not been here." Freya cried and cried. Wherever she went she left tears of amber behind her, trailing her path of sorrow. The trees ceased to bloom, the flowers withered and died, and a sheet of glimmering snow covered the grounds as Freya passed by, so cold was her heart.

For many months she met with the same answer until she was far away from her home at a little place in the sunny south. There she found Odin sitting beneath a myrtle tree. When Freya spotted him, her heart leapt. Finally, finally her heart burst open with joy at seeing the man she loved. The myrtle tree immediately blossomed and was covered with a thousand flowers, so contagious was Freya's joy.

Odin was overjoyed to see her, for all his adventures were meaningless without his true love to share them with. Hand in hand once more, the two lovers made their way back home, and wherever they went the grass grew, the flowers bloomed, and the birds sang. All of nature rejoiced with Freya's happiness, just as it had mourned with her sorrow.

At first glance, this love story may seem as if Freya is unable to live without a man in her life. She throws everything away to go off in search of Odin. On a deeper level this story illustrates the changing of the seasons. Odin is the god of war, storms, magic, inspiration, and the underworld. His relationship with Freya is interdependent—they need each other to produce the different seasons. When they are together their union produces the spring and summer months, and when they are apart their separation causes fall and winter.

Many cultures have similar seasonal myths, like the Greek story of Demeter the fertility goddess and her daughter, Persephone. When Persephone was abducted by Hades, the god of the underworld, Demeter was so upset she stopped everything from growing. Finally a bargain was struck. Persephone spent part of the year in the underworld with Hades; this produced the winter months. Then she spent part of the year on earth with her mother, thus producing spring and summer.

....

Goddess Workout

Do you think Freya overreacted when Odin left her?

Have you ever been so in love that you were tempted to drop everything and run off after a guy you liked?

If so, what was the result of your actions?

About Freya

Freya is a goddess of fertility and creativity, as you can see by the fact that all of nature blooms in her presence. Her moods have a direct impact on the weather, just as your moods have a direct impact on your environment. She rode in her chariot with her brother Frey, which was drawn by a golden-haired boar. She scattered fruits and flowers to gladden the heart of all humankind.

Freya and Frey were held in such high honor that even today their names are still used for "master" and "mistress" in the North. There were many goddess temples dedicated to Freya in the Norse lands—Sweden, Norway, Denmark, and Iceland. She was the goddess of sexuality and her special day, Freya's day, is Friday. Lovers often say prayers to her and she will give them her blessing. Many love songs have been composed in her honor. On special occasions it was customary to drink a toast to Freya's health. As Scandinavia became Christianized, this custom was transferred to Mary and to St. Gertrude.

Freya is a personification of the Earth. She has a special affection for the fairies, who she loves to watch dancing in the moonbeams. She would give the fairies her daintiest flowers and sweetest honey as tokens of her adoration.

Air People

People who have a lot of air energy in them, like Freya, have certain characteristics. Physically they are tall and thin, with a narrow skeletal frame. They may suffer from physical conditions such as dry skin, arthritis, psoriasis, and dandruff. They are very mentally active. They love to think about stuff and analyze it. They tend to hold on to things intellectually rather than just letting it go. Air people can have a hard time letting anything go mentally. When used appropriately, air people can focus their imagination and use it to create amazing things. When used destructively, air people can be the world's greatest worrywarts. They tend to live in their heads rather than their hearts.

They can be very argumentative and rational and have a hard time getting into their emotions. Their arguments often begin with the words "I think," "I believe," or "I know."

Keeping Air In Balance

The element of air is important in your emotional body because it helps you to think rationally. Air helps you to let go of things that no longer serve you and to make a fresh start. Air keeps your mind fresh and your life fresh. It keeps you moving when your life falls into a rut. Air is the motivating force in change.

Too Little Air

Too little air in your life makes you unable to think clearly. People without much air become stuck in a rut. They are very rigid in their ideals and in their beliefs. Nothing can sway them from their viewpoint. They are argumentative to the point of being obnoxious, and always like to have the last word. Do you know anyone like this? Too little air can lead to a person feeling stagnated and can make them depressed.

Too Much Air

What do you think of when you think of a space cadet? Well, that is someone with too *much* air! People who have an awful lot of air in their demeanor are spacey, impractical, and often infuriatingly vague. They are impulsive and sometimes act irrationally without thinking about the consequences of their actions. Sometimes when the mind is so overactive it can lead to paranoia, where you hear voices in your head. (This is not the same as clairaudience.)

How to Get More Air

If you feel like you don't have enough air in your life, and you feel like you are in a bit of a rut, there are several things you can do to increase your air levels:

- Take a hike up a mountain

- Breathe deeply—drinking in air automatically increases the amount of air in you!

- Do something differently—walk home a different way from school, get up at a different time, read a new book

What If You Have Too Much Air?

If you feel like you are sometimes a spacey person and want to get more grounded, all you need to do is increase the amount of earth in your life. To do this, try:

- Eating root vegetables, like carrots or potatoes

- Lying on the ground for twenty minutes

- Doing something totally in your body, like running or swimming

- Not reading for an entire week

Use Your Mind

In many cultures, the mind is associated with the element of air. Your mind is one of your greatest tools and you can use it to affect great change in your life. How do you use your mind most often? Do you use it to tell yourself scary things or kind things? Is your mind a fun place to hang out or a horrible place?

Worry is one of the worst habits you can use your mind for. Why? Because worry never changes a thing. All worry does is make you feel bad about stuff. It can even paralyze you to the point where you feel incapable of changing things.

However, if you are a worrywart, I have good news for you. Here are some steps to follow.

How to Break the Worry Habit

1) Remember, worrying is just a habit, and a bad habit at that. You became a worrier by worrying a lot, and you can break the habit just like you can break any bad habit. You break the worry habit by choosing to think about something else.

2) Faith and optimism are the opposite to worry, so when a worry thought pops into your head, immediately replace it with an optimistic one. Say out loud: "Go away, stupid thought" when you think a worry thought.

3) When you start to worry, say: "Everything will be okay," "I am always divinely guided and divinely protected," and "The Goddess is taking care of it."

4) Practice saying constructive things instead of negative things. Instead of saying "Today is just not my day," say "I'm going to enjoy this day whatever turns up—it is all part of life's experiences." Instead of saying "I'm never going to be able to pass this exam," say "I am going to do my best and do whatever I can to make sure I pass this exam."

5) Ask empowering questions. Instead of asking "Why does this always happen to me?" ask "What can I do to move through this?" Ask questions that propel you forward instead of keeping you stuck.

6) Don't hang out with other worrywarts. Worriers thrive on more worry. The worse the story, the more they love it! If people are having a conversation about how terrible everything is, refuse to be drawn into it. Say to yourself, "Well, that might be true for them, but it is certainly not true for me."

7) Remember that every problem can be solved.

8) Use your mind in a way that enhances your life.

Important Points to Remember

- It is *your* mind; you can use it how you want.

- Your mind can be your best friend or your worst enemy.

- You can tell yourself horror stories or happy endings.

- You are the only thinker in your mind—no one else.

- What *you* think of you is what counts.

- You can think whatever you like about yourself, your life, your abilities, your future, your past—anything.

What are you thinking about today?

Air Magic

The Air Goddess is the best goddess to go to when you have any problems in the area of arguments, feeling bored or restless, or when you have a condition in your life that you wish would magically disappear.

The types of magic that are specific to the Air Goddess are prayers, incantations, affirmations, and meditations. These techniques all deal with the mind or with the breath, which falls into the realm of the Air Goddess.

How to Deal with Argumentative People

The Air Goddess can help you with arguments you are having with others. People usually argue because they feel misunderstood or they are trying to get their point across. Arguments can escalate very quickly if people start insulting each other, name-calling, or trying to get one-up over the other person. Words flung in an argument can hurt deeply and be hard to overcome later.

The next time you find yourself in an argument with someone, try the following steps so you can communicate clearly and come to a better understanding of the other person. All of us want to be understood, and learning good communication skills is a great asset.

First, Ask the Air Goddess for Help

Let's say you are right smack in the middle of an argument. Stop, take a deep breath, and say a quick prayer to the Air Goddess. Ask her for clarity, to be able to communicate effectively, and to give you insight into how the other person is feeling.

Listen from Your Heart

Concentrate on what the other person is saying. Sometimes when we fight, we try to drown out the other person's thoughts, opinions, or ideas with our own. We spend more time trying to get our point across than listening to what the other person is saying. Open your heart and use all your skills of understanding and compassion to hear what the other person is saying. Listen to what you think their heart is trying to tell you. What do you think they are feeling?

Talk from your heart, too. Often when we argue, we get muddled up in talking about external things instead of saying what we really feel. My husband always used to accuse me of doing this. Instead of saying I was feeling overwhelmed by all the stuff I had to do that day, I would pick an argument with him about something stupid. When I started talking from my heart and sharing my true feelings, we had a lot less arguments.

To talk from your heart, share your feelings. Start sentences with "I feel like . . ."

....
Goddess Workout

Sometime during the day today, ask a person that you usually don't communicate very well with "How's it going?" Listen to them from your heart and use these skills to see if you are understanding what they are saying. Tune in to how the person is feeling. Talk to them from your heart, too.

PAY ATTENTION TO THE OTHER PERSON

Use the skills of a good warrior and tune into what is going on with the other person. Look at their body language, and listen to the tone of their words as well as listening to what they are saying. If you can look beyond their words and observe what their body is telling you and what their tone of voice is saying, you will get a lot of valuable information that will tell you how they are feeling.

USE MIRRORING TO SEE IF YOU ARE HEARING WHAT THEY ARE SAYING

Mirroring is a counseling technique that teaches you to listen effectively. Pretend you are a mirror. Whatever you hear the other person saying, you mirror back to them to make sure you understand what they are saying or feeling. You repeat in your own words what you think they mean. For example, let's say you are having an argument with your mom. You want to go to the movies with your friends and this is what she says:

Mom says heatedly: "No, you can't go to the movies; it's a school night and you need to stay home!"

You: "It sounds like you are kind of angry about me wanting to go to the movies."

Mom: "You bet I am! You spend far too much time out with your friends instead of doing your homework."

You: "Are you worried that my grades are suffering?"

Mom: "Yes."

Now we are getting somewhere. With mirroring you discover the *real* reasons people are upset. Let's say you had an argument without using mirroring or trying to understand what the other person was feeling. It could have gone like this:

Mom says heatedly: "No, you can't go to the movies; it's a school night and you need to stay home!"

You: "That's not fair! You never let me go anywhere. All the other girls' moms let them go out."

Mom: "I don't care what the other moms do, I'm not them."

You: "No, you are way meaner than them!"

Mom: "You are not going out, and that is final."

What has been solved from this scenario? Nothing. You both end up feeling rotten. In the first scenario you have a better understanding of what your mom is feeling, and this gives you room to see if you can negotiate.

LOOK FOR A SOLUTION INSTEAD OF TRYING TO PROVE YOU ARE RIGHT

Put yourself on the same side as your "opponent" and see if you can come up with a solution or a compromise that will work for both of you. For example, in the situation above, a good place to go from the first scenario, now that you know your mom is concerned about your schoolwork, would be:

You: "Well, how would you feel if I got all my homework done before I went to the movies?"

Mom: "Well, what about studying? Do you have any tests coming up?"

You: "I don't have any tests tomorrow but I have a history paper that is due on Monday. I could finish my homework and spend thirty minutes studying, too."

Mom: "That sounds like a good idea."

You: "So if I get finished before the movies and show you what I have done, can I go?"

Mom: "I don't see why not."

In that example, you both win. Mom has the satisfaction of knowing you are on track with your schoolwork, and you have a situation you can work with. Get all your homework done and you can go out.

....

Goddess Workout

Try to come up with a solution where you both gain something the next time you have a disagreement with someone. Pray to the Air Goddess to inspire you with creative solutions. Brainstorm, don't give up, and think up as many solutions as you can, no matter how silly or far-fetched. You are bound to come up with one that will work.

IF YOU ARE GETTING MAD, TAKE SOME TIME OUT

If your temperature reaches boiling point in the middle of an argument, take some time out. Nothing can be resolved when you are fuming mad. Best to go for a walk around the block and blow off some steam before trying to sort things out.

How to Make Problems Magically Disappear

Have you ever wished you could make your problems magically disappear in a puff of smoke? Well, with a little assistance from the Air Goddess, you can.

Find a place to sit down to do this exercise, and close your eyes.

Think about a problem, a person, or a situation that is troubling you and that you wish was no longer a part of your life. You can think about a hurt, a resentment, or an injury instead, if that is more applicable. Choose a color that you feel represents the situation. Now see it as a big cloud before you. The cloud contains the person, situation, or hurt you want to fade from your life experience. The cloud is the color you have chosen.

Now see the cloud shrinking before your very eyes. A large gust of wind comes along and lifts it up into the sky. It moves farther and farther away from you, getting smaller and smaller as it does. You watch it move until it is no longer in sight.

Say a prayer: "This (condition, person, etc.) now fades from my life. I am in the enchanted circle of the Goddess's love and protection."

Now you have to act as if the condition is no longer in your life. This means no longer talking about it and no longer thinking about it. If you find it pops into your mind, then you must immediately replace it with a thought about something else.

If it was a bad experience that you want to be free of, one thing you can do is pretend it was a nightmare. When thoughts about it arise, say "Okay, that happened, it is in the past and *this* is what I want to be experiencing now." Then focus on what you do want to be experiencing.

With magic you can make the good things in your life larger and the bad things smaller. It is all a question of where you rest your attention.

Freya's Glamour

- Pastel clothing

- Gold jewelry

- Bells

- Sparkly gold eye shadow

- Her makeup is light and fresh

- Her clothes are flowing and delicate, like a spring flower

- Citrus perfumes, such as lemon or orange blossom

- Yellow and apricot foods

Makeup

Her makeup is light and fresh, like a pale peach lipstick and shimmery yellow eye shadow. Use a light foundation or tinted moisturizer and smooth over your face. Apply the yellow eye shadow from the lash line of the upper lids to just above the eye creases. Take a liquid blue eyeliner and apply across the lash line of the upper lid. Use a natural brown pencil eyeliner on the lower line. Blend a sheeny purple eye shadow over the outer corners of the upper lid.

Use a peach-based cream blush on the apple of your cheeks—just a very sheer touch of color. Then apply a peachy pink crème lipstick to your lips.

Wear a perfume with a citrus base, such as lemon, lime, or orange.

Clothing

Anything yellow, light, or airy. Choose clothes that are light in texture, like a chiffon skirt or a silk blouse. Spring is a wonderful season for buying floral clothes so one suggestion is to wear a long, flowing, floral dress. Think spring, think light and airy, and you can't go wrong.

Ceremony

The Air Goddess rules the realm of flight, so for this ceremony you are going to take a journey to another land. To a shaman this is known as a shamanic journey to the otherworlds.

What you will need is some music that makes you feel very relaxed. Get into your Air Goddess gears, put on the music, and then lie down on your bed.

Now begin to relax your whole body. Start with your legs. Feel your legs get lighter and lighter; imagine you are floating on a cloud and your body feels incredibly light. A gentle wind blows over you, cleansing away all the frustrations, irritations, and worry from your day. Now your attention moves up into your torso; feel your torso become incredibly relaxed. Your torso feels lighter and lighter. Now move up to your head and shoulders; they, too, now feel incredibly relaxed. Your whole body feels wonderful, as if you are floating on air.

Now imagine a small opening at the top of your head. You see a white sparkly funnel placed in the opening. The Air Goddess now comes toward you and you feel her energy enter the funnel like a whirlwind. It breezes down through your head, cleansing your mind of all outworn thoughts and beliefs. It sweeps through your entire body, this purifying wind, clearing away any negativity. You feel the energy of the Air Goddess illuminating you, renewing you, and you feel so very, very light. You feel fresh with the sparkle of spring.

Now you see a chariot coming toward you. It is a beautiful golden chariot emblazoned with precious jewels in ruby and amber. Sitting in the chariot is Freya, dressed in a long, shimmery, ice-yellow gown. There is a sparkling golden crown on her head that glitters at you. You close your eyes for a second because the light is so bright. Freya motions for you to come forward. You do so and climb into the chariot to sit beside her. Now the chariot takes off into the sky. You feel the energy of air all around you as your body swirls and dips and rises with the motion of the chariot.

You see stars and planets whiz by you as you travel farther and farther. Everything becomes a blur in your vision, as you are going so fast.

Freya is taking you into the future. Six months from now, you see your life. What are you doing? What are you wearing? How do you look? You see all the changes that have taken place in your life. You see all the old bad habits you have left behind and all the new healthy ones you have acquired.

"I will help you acquire this, one day at a time," Freya promises.

"You must be willing to shed your old thoughts and your old habits as a snake sheds its skin," Freya says.

"Together we will renew your mind, renew your life, and plant new seeds so that your life will bear much fruit."

You sit and talk with Freya for a while about what you need to let go of and what steps you need to take so your life will bear much fruit in the next six months.

When you are ready, you thank Freya and she brings you back down to your room. You feel her power course through your body like a gentle wind, renewing you and refreshing you. You are able to look at your life from a new perspective and you feel energized.

Freya's Tasks for You

- Get up early one morning and greet the Air Goddess at dawn. Ask her to bless your day with inspiration and clear thinking.

- Practice using good communication skills this week in your conversations. Observe other peoples' conversations (be an eavesdropper!) and see if you can hear where they are using good skills and not-so-good skills.

- Practice listening with your eyes, ears, and heart to what people are saying with their bodies, their tone of voice, and see if you can figure out what they are feeling. Watch a sitcom with the sound off for ten minutes and guess what emotions are being displayed by body action alone.

- Be the Air Goddess one day this week. Write down your experiences in your goddess journal.

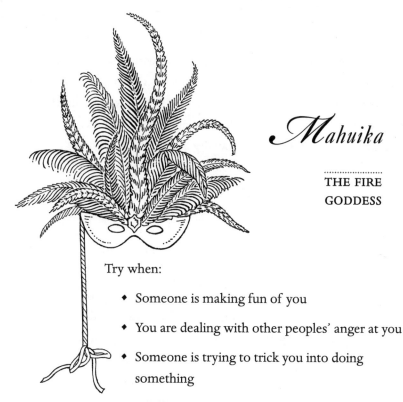

Mahuika

**THE FIRE
GODDESS**

Try when:

- Someone is making fun of you

- You are dealing with other peoples' anger at you

- Someone is trying to trick you into doing
  something

- You are consumed with jealousy

- You want to increase your confidence

The Fire Goddess is feisty and unrestrained. She is a mover
and a shaker, not one to sit on the shelf gathering dust. Her
motto is "I don't wait for the action, I *make* the action." She is
exciting and dynamic to be around. She carries a flaming
spear in her outstretched arms. Her spear represents focused
passion, the power of determination.

The Fire Goddess does not take "no" for an answer. She is
the one who will make a way where there is no way. She is a
trailblazer who lights the way for others to follow. If you have
a cause you want to take up or a path you must forge into unknown territory, the Fire Goddess is the one who can light
your way.

Mentally she will give you the courage of your convictions. She will strengthen your resolve so you can take effective action to obtain victory in all areas of your life. She will give you endurance and stamina, and teach you how to be steadfast in your commitments. She will give you the gift of experience that comes from taking action, for it is only from doing so that you can discover your true abilities.

The Fire Goddess will give you the confidence to undertake many tasks you never before thought possible. She will teach you how to express yourself in the world. You will learn how to act on the inspirations you received from the Air Goddess.

244

Mahuika (pronounced *ma-who-ee-ka*) is the Maori goddess of fire. When I was a little girl I loved the story of how Mahuika gave Maui fire, although some people say Maui tricked the Goddess into giving it to him. Goddesses, however, cannot be tricked into doing anything they don't want to do. Anytime they do something that involves a trick, it is usually a rite of passage or initiation for the person involved.

Fire was made in ancient Maori times by rubbing two sticks together. When I was small my friends and I would try to make fire in this way. In Maori times, fire was imperative for cooking food. Food was cooked in a *hangi*, which is a hole dug into the ground where food wrapped in flax is placed to cook slowly for several hours. Fish, meat, birds, and root vegetables are all cooked this way. The food is delicious, filled with flavors that come from being lovingly prepared and painstakingly cooked. Today Maori people still have a hangi anytime there is a reason to celebrate, just as your family might have a barbecue.

I am part Maori. I come from the Ngati Raukawa tribe in Otaki, New Zealand. My people were ruled by the seasons. They were warriors, a race who would eat their enemies so they could say, "I've got your great, great grandfather in my *puku* (stomach)!" They were carvers, artists, weavers, fisherfolk, and storytellers. I remember my great aunt bicycling to the beach early in the morning with her huge net over her shoulder right up until she was in her eighties to catch whitebait to eat.

Each tribe lived on a *Marae* (village) in wooden huts raised up off the ground. Their lives were filled with family, ancestors, magic, and myth. The spirit world is very important to the Maori.

Today if you visit New Zealand you can go into a Marae and see the beautiful wall hangings and carvings that adorn the buildings and tell the story of each family.

Mahuika's Story

How she gave fire to Maui and the people of Aotearoa (New Zealand)

Once upon a time, a long, long time ago, there was a mischievous young man named Maui. One day he decided to put out all the fires in the world just to see what would happen. So after all the people in his village had gone to bed for the night, when the moon was high in the sky and the air was still and quiet, Maui snuck around his village and extinguished every single fire. He knew that the only way to get fire was from his ancestress, Mahuika, the fire goddess.

When morning came, Maui was anxious to see what would happen, so as soon as the sun shined his rosy tip above the mountain, Maui called out to his *pononga*, his servants:

"I'm starving, quick—cook me some food and bring it to me, for my stomach aches from hunger!"

One of his servants hurried outside to cook the food and found the fire was out. He went to the neighboring house but there was no fire there either, so he ran to the next house. No fire. On and on he ran until he had visited every home in the Marae. Not one single fire was there.

When Maui's mother heard what had happened, she called her servants to her. "Quickly, now, you must go visit my great ancestress Mahuika. For she is the goddess of fire and will provide a light for us—she carries fire in each of her fingernails and each of her toenails."

The servants shuffled and shook. None of them had any desire to go to Mahuika, for they had heard of her fierceness. And they had no desire to see the

Goddess with the blazing fingernails and blazing toenails. The sacred elders of the tribe gathered together and commanded the servants to go, but still they refused. Not even the threat of severe punishment was enough to make them change their minds.

Maui had been waiting for all this. And he called out to his mother, "All right, then, I will go! Show me the way!"

"You must follow this road, Maui," said his mother. "But for goodness' sake, don't be playing any of your tricks on Mahuika, for she does not suffer fools."

However, Maui had other ideas, and off he set in search of the great fire goddess Mahuika.

Well it didn't take long for him to find her. She was a tall, striking woman, with long, wavy brown hair and skin the color of fertile soil. Her eyes were dark as burning coals and indeed they seemed to burn right through him as she turned her gaze upon him.

"What have we here?" she demanded. Tiny sparks of fire fell from her skin with each movement of her body.

"Great ancestress," said Maui. "Our fires have gone out and you must give us more, for surely the people in my land will die with no heat and no fire to cook our food."

Mahuika rose to her full height. She towered over Maui. "Aue!" she hurled the words at him with enough force to throw him backwards. "Who are you?"

"I have come from the land where the wind blows upon me," he replied, pulling himself up.

"Well, then," she began. "You are my grandchild." She stepped forward and brought her face down level with him, and searched him with her scorching eyes. "Why do you visit me, young Maui?"

"Because all the fires in our village have died during the night and we need you to give us more fire."

"Well, then," she repeated, "here you go," and she pulled off the fingernail of her *koiti*, her little finger. As she drew it out, fire blazed from it and she handed it to Maui. He was impressed but tried not to show it, and headed off. But as soon as he was out of Mahuika's sight, he put the fire out and returned to her.

"The fire you gave me has gone out, Grandmother," he said. "You must give me some more."

So Mahuika pulled the fire from her *manawa*, her third finger, and gave it to him. Maui went off again and then wet the fiery fingernail and told Mahuika he had fallen into a stream.

Mahuika gave him the fiery fingernail from her *mapere*, her middle finger, and he did the same thing until Mahuika had given him all her fingernails and toenails except for one. By now she could see that Maui was trying to trick her into giving him all her fire.

When he came back this time begging for fire, Mahuika turned to him, her feet firmly planted on the ground, her eyes blazing, and her voice low and deadly. "You want fire, little one?" she whispered. "WELL, HERE IT IS, THEN!" she shrieked and threw the fire with all her might so that it spread like hot lava upon the ground. It chased Maui, it singed his toes, it climbed into the trees.

Maui ran for his life with the fire chasing him, consuming the land in its wake. Pretty soon the forests were aflame and the surrounding lands were ablaze, too. Maui changed himself into a hawk to escape the fire and tried to soar above the flames, but the fire leapt higher and higher and scorched his feathers, which is why even today the *karearea* (hawk) has flaming feathers. He saw a lake and plunged into it, but was nearly boiled alive for the fire had already heated the waters. Everywhere the land was alight.

Maui was exhausted. He cried out to the sky, "Let there be rain!"

Great clouds appeared and Tawhiri, the god of storms, sent a sprinkling of rain, which got stronger and stronger until everything was drenched.

Mahuika had been watching from her home and now she commanded the fire to find shelter in the trees before it perished from the oncoming storm. So the fire crawled within the bark of the hinau, the rata, the totara, and other native trees of New Zealand.

And Maui returned to his village and was shamed by his elders for not bringing fire.

"How will we eat?" wept his mother. "With what shall we cook? And when the sky is frozen with dark clouds and the snow cloaks the ground, with what shall we warm ourselves?"

Maui, however, was not one for learning lessons. "What do I care?" he snapped. "Do you think I will be different because of this? Certainly not! I will be just the same forever!"

His father gazed quietly at him. "You alone choose whether you will live or die. We cannot make that choice for you, Maui. Your choices, be they impetuous or be they wise, are yours alone."

And then Mahuika came down to the village and showed the people how she had hidden her fire in the trees. She taught them how to call forth fire for themselves by rubbing a digging stick in a piece of grooved wood. And so Mahuika gave her people the gift of fire forever.

The Fire Goddess

There are many myths from different cultures that describe the Goddess as the keeper of the flame. Just like Bridget was the keeper of the sacred flame in Celtic mythology, so, too, is Mahuika the keeper of the flame in Maori mythology. In this way women are seen as the keepers of the hearth and of spiritual power, for in ancient times fire was a metaphor for spiritual power. In various stories a teacher will pass on spiritual understanding to a student through the form of a flame taken from one great fire.

Fire People

People who have a lot of fire in them generally have intense, penetrating eyes. They tend to be slender, as their metabolism is high and quickly burns up the food they eat. Their skin can become flushed quickly and they can have a ruddy complexion. They often have a predisposition to dilated capillaries, which makes their faces appear red and blotchy.

Fire people are fidgety and get angry quickly. "Temperamental" is a good word to describe them. However, they are also quick to take action and they are highly motivated to get stuff done. Fire people are competitive. They think quickly and act quickly. They take action in an emergency rather than panic. When their anger does flare up, it dies down quickly, and they don't often hold grudges, although some fire people hold on to resentments and let them smolder for a very long time.

Fire people have strong egos. They tend to be very assertive and confident. They often excel at sports and debating. They make enthusiastic plans and are passionate about their ideas.

Keeping Fire In Balance

Watch how you use your fire. Fire is the quality that gives you enthusiasm and passion. One mistake people make when using their inner fire is to get very enthusiastic about a project and then run around telling everyone of their great plans. All the energy goes into the telling rather than the doing. So when it is time to put your project together, your enthusiasm and inner fire has died down and you don't have any motivation left to actually do it.

Fire is also the quality of anger, jealousy, and rage. When fire has no outlet, it smolders and burns. A fire that is fueled and stoked can burn out of control, blazing everything in its path, just as anger that is not kept in check can quickly turn into rage and destroy everything in its sight.

Too Little Fire

Too little fire makes you unmotivated, depressed, and lethargic. When you don't have enough fire, you find it hard to get motivated and to be active. You may feel like a couch potato, and spend your time playing video games or watching TV. Challenges seem overwhelming and you may find your confidence waning. Little things can seem like a big deal. You may be frightened of any kind of conflict and avoid it at all costs, and be threatened by bullies or aggressive people.

Too Much Fire

When you have too much fire, you will feel restless, hyperactive, or irritable. Lots of fire can make a person self-centered and uncaring. You may be extremely competitive and envious of others. Jealousy may be a problem for you. You may find yourself snapping at people for no reason or overreacting with anger at the slightest provocation.

How to Get More Fire

If you want to raise the amount of fire in your system, eat hot, spicy foods. Wear red or orange. Eat foods from the sun like oranges, pineapples, carrots, peppers, and tomatoes. Wear red stones like garnets or rubies. Exercise with an aerobic exercise—anything that will get your heart pounding. Spend some time out in the sun (wearing sunscreen, of course).

What If You Have Too Much Fire?

Eat cooling foods that contain a lot of water, like cucumber or lettuce. Drink lots of water. Avoid spicy foods. Do a relaxing type of exercise, like yoga or meditation. Spend time outside under the moon to decrease your yang energy and increase your yin. Wear blue or green-colored clothes. Exercise aerobically every day first thing in the morning or in the evening to burn off the excess fire, then have a cool shower.

Women in Maori Society

Women have a special place in Maori society. Actually all people do—old people and young people are all honored for their contributions: old people for their wisdom and insight and young people for their energy. However, women are the sacred gatekeepers in Maori tradition. When you go to a Marae, it is the woman who decides whether you can enter or not.

A Marae is a Maori meeting place. In the olden days people used to live in the Marae just like the Native Americans lived in pueblos. The Marae was enclosed by a wooden fence to keep intruders out. When my mother was a child her family lived one block away from their Marae. The Marae is the heart-center of the tribe. It is a place to gather for special occasions and festivities, as well as for funerals (*tangis*), important meetings, weddings, and spiritual nourishment. Being allowed to visit a Marae is a great honor.

When visitors arrive at a Marae, they must wait outside until they are asked to enter. There are four steps that take place when you go into a Marae:

1. A challenge is issued by the tribe

2. The challenge is accepted by the visiting party

3. A *Kai Karanga* (sacred caller) issues an invitation of welcome

4. A woman from the visiting party accepts the welcome and the visitors move forward

Sometimes steps one and two are left out, depending on the situation, but for all formal occasions they are included. Sometimes three challenges are made instead of one. This is for a very formal occasion, like when the prime minister goes to visit, or if there is reason to believe the visitors have not come in peace.

The visitors wait at the gate until they are ushered inside the Marae. Then the challenge (*Wero*) is given while the guests stand near the gate. They are not allowed to proceed forward until the proper protocol has taken place.

The Wero is an old tradition that tribes would give to determine if their visitors came in peace or in war. A man issues the Wero. His purpose is to intimidate the visitors by his fierceness and strength. The challenger dances a fierce war dance and makes scary faces at the visitors, and he may also boast of his ancestors' conquests and the prowess of his tribe. Then he places a spear at the feet of the guests. If he points the spear toward the visitors, he is saying that he thinks they have come to make trouble. If he lays the spear alongside the visitors, he is showing he believes they have come in peace, and if he throws it at them, they had better run for their lives!

The head of the visitors then picks up the spear, signaling they have come in peace. This tradition is performed without any physical contact between the visitors and the tribe. It is part of an ancient tradition where the challenger would be watching his guests using his spiritual senses as well as his physical ones to pick up their intent.

The spear was placed for two reasons: one, as a silent invitation to the guests to come into the Marae, and two, to give the guests an opportunity to state their business and to resolve any differences peacefully while acknowledging that some challenging words may be spoken. It was a way of saying, "Okay, you are here, you may proceed, we understand that you may have a bone to pick with us, but let's sort it out as amicably as possible." By picking up the spear, the guests are saying "Okay" back.

The next step is for the Kai Karanga to extend an invitation of welcome to the visitors. The Kai Karanga is always a woman and it is a great honor to hold this position. You are the sacred gatekeeper of the tribe. You hold the spiritual key of entry for guests to visit. If there is no Kai Karanga present in the Marae, the guests must wait until one shows up. They cannot proceed without being issued this sacred invitation.

Maori is a magical language that is still spoken today. Hebrew and Hawaiian are two more magical languages that are also still spoken. Unlike English, words in magical languages have many different layers of meaning. They can have spiritual meaning, emotional meaning, and a literal meaning.

For example, if I said to my grandmother, "I am going to go fishing at the ocean," she could interpret it in three different ways:

1. I am going to go to the ocean and get some fish (this is the literal meaning)

2. I am going to go to the ocean to feed my spirit and enjoy the beauty of the day (this is the emotional meaning)

3. I am going to go visit the Goddess of Water to seek answers to questions that I have about my life (this is the spiritual meaning)

So when the Kai Karanga gives her call, she is extending a literal invitation of welcome into the Marae. Plus she is issuing a spiritual invitation and an emotional invitation—a heart salutation. She is saying, in essence, "We as a tribe honor you, we honor you, we honor your ancestors, we honor your tribe and your divinity. Welcome from our hearts, welcome from our spirits, and welcome from our ancestors."

Words are sacred in the Maori tradition. They are believed to have great power. Words can create or they can destroy. They are powerful weapons and must be used carefully. With words you can cut, wound, heal, lull to sleep, enchant, mesmerize, seduce, and motivate.

....
Goddess Workout

Imagine words are your sacred weapon. How have you been using them lately? Pay attention to the way you use them for the next couple of days. Practice using them to achieve a desired result—to create trust or to motivate or uplift others. Write a list of ten ways you can use words.

When the Kai Karanga calls her invitation, she is creating a sacred pathway into the Marae for the guests to walk through in safety and in trust. She is setting up her intent—a pathway in the spirit realms—through the use of her words.

A *karanga* (sacred call) goes something like this:

> *Welcome, welcome*
>
> *Visitors from far away*
>
> *Come forward*
>
> *Onto our sacred Marae*
>
> *Bring with you your ancestors' spirits*
>
> *That we may greet them too*
>
> *Welcome to the Marae*
>
> *Of our people*

This call is very meaningful because it is the first words spoken to the visitors.

Then the visitors must answer with their own greeting, and only a woman can return the call. Once the proper steps have been taken, then other members of the tribe can speak. But it is always the women who must set up the verbal exchange first, otherwise the guests cannot enter the Marae.

Plus women have the power to end a man's speech on the Marae. If a man has been speaking for too long, a woman elder may stand and begin singing a *waiata* (song) to cut him off! The man has no choice but to finish speaking and join in the song. Another way a woman can stop a man from speaking is to walk in front of him while he is talking. This signals he must stop talking and sit down. Of course it would have to be an extreme situation for a woman elder to do this, but she does have the power to do it. Men don't!

There are no formal lessons to teach women to become a Kai Karanga. This skill is learned from years of going onto the Marae and watching and listening to what is done. Girls generally do not Kai Karanga while they have a grandmother, mother, or older sister still alive. My great aunt was a Kai Karanga for our tribe before she died. When my family went into the Marae for my mother's funeral, my great aunt gave the karanga to the guests who would not normally be on a Marae.

How to Use Your Anger to Take Charge of Your Life

Like Mahuika, you can direct your inner fire and your anger so it will serve you well.

Anger is an ally. It will teach you many lessons about how you want to be treated, what you think is fair, and how to stand up for injustice. Anger prompts you to take action to ensure justice takes place. Anger is cathartic. It can point you in a direction that empowers you.

The difference between anger and rage is that rage is violent, rage threatens to destroy, rage is anger out of control. Rage is the kind of vehemence where you want to destroy everything in sight—where you just lash out and don't care who or what gets hurt in the process. When you express rage, there is very often a big mess to clean up afterwards.

Anger is helpful, rage is hurtful.

Expressing your anger makes you feel strong and powerful. Expressing rage makes you feel depleted and out of control. Anger seeks to find an active solution, rage seeks destruction.

What Is Your Anger Telling You?

Anger is a sign that you need to make some changes. Either you need to put some boundaries in place with people in your life or you need to stand up for yourself. Start speaking your truth and see what happens. Anger often builds up when we agree to do things that we don't really want to do or feel like we are being treated unfairly.

Close your eyes and ask your anger what message it is giving you. Write it down on a piece of paper. Ask, "Anger, what are you trying to tell me?" Write whatever comes out for ten minutes without stopping. Then ask, "Anger, what actions do I need to take to remedy this situation?" Write for another ten minutes about whatever comes up.

....
Goddess Workout

Who are you most angry at right now?

What are you angry at them for?

When have you stood up for yourself and how did it feel?

If you feel frightened of standing up for yourself and often let people walk all over you, ask Mahuika to help you. Ask her to light the fires of justice and courage within you. Make a point of standing up for yourself the next time you feel belittled in some way. Imagine Mahuika with you, helping you.

Coping with Rage:
What to Do When It Is Out of Control

What do you do if you find yourself exploding way out of proportion to a situation—when you feel rage rising like a volcano from your stomach and threatening to explode over everything like hot lava?

Well, first, you need to do something to release the heated feelings in a safe way, and then you need to explore where all the rage is coming from. If rage is a common experience for you, seek the help of your school counselor.

Ways to Dilute Rage

- Put on some loud rock music and do a *haka* (a Maori war dance). Imagine all your ancestors are standing behind you. Dance your rage out of your body. Close your eyes and listen to your body—what is the anger telling you? How does your body want to move? Make vocal sounds if you can.

- Go for a swim in the ocean. If you don't have an ocean, a swimming pool or cold shower will do. Stay in the water until you feel the rage leaving your body. Drenching yourself with cool water is one of the quickest ways to extinguish flaming rage.

- Play a game of racquetball by yourself or with a friend. Slam the ball against the wall and put all your energy into each shot. Feel the fire coming down your arms and extending out of your fingertips, just like Mahuika.

- Each morning say a prayer to Mahuika that your inner fire may guide you and warm you and light the way for you for that day. Ask her to help you temper your fire so that it does not burn out of control and hurt you or anyone else.

What to Do if You Are Fighting with Your Best Friend

Fighting with your best friend sucks. I know—I have been fighting with my best friend (my husband!) today. I have tons of work to do and I'm having trouble concentrating because all I can think about is the mean things we said to each other and how bad I feel.

When you're fighting with your best friend, it can feel like your whole world is turned upside-down. If it's a really horrible fight you may feel scared that your whole friendship is on the line. Thoughts like "What if she won't talk to me ever again?" or "What if she wants to stop being my friend?" can cross your mind. You may go from feeling so mad that you think you never want to see her again to feeling scared that your friendship is over and she may never want to see you again.

Remember, underneath great anger is great hurt; you need to take a moment to look through the anger and see what kind of hurt lies underneath. Ask yourself "What am I hurting about?" Then ask, "What might my friend be hurting about?" Take some time out to sort out your feelings and get into a space where you can see things from a bigger perspective. Here are some tips I find helpful that may help you, too.

Take Time Out

If you are arguing a lot or in the middle of a fight that is escalating, stop and say, "I need a breather. Let's talk about this later." Remove yourself from the situation and take care of yourself. If you are feeling mad, do something that will blow off some steam—go for a run, put on some loud music and dance for fifteen minutes, or take a cool shower. After the anger has dissipated, journal about your feelings— what you are cross about and why, how you are feeling underneath, and think about how your best friend might be feeling. Let all your feelings out on paper.

Talk with Your Goddess Self

Close your eyes and get in touch with your inner goddess. See your goddess self as larger than you and larger than the fight. Ask your inner goddess for guidance on how to deal with the situation. Ask one of the goddesses in this book for help; you might choose Kuan Yin to bring compassion into your heart, or Mary to help you gain clarity on the situation. Ask as many goddesses as you like and see them in your imagination standing around you encircling you with love. Write down in your goddess journal any ideas or thoughts that come to you. Have a conversation with the Goddess on paper asking her questions and writing the answers.

Make a Heart Connection with Your Friend

Close your eyes again and in your imagination see your inner goddess. Now imagine your friend standing before you and see her as her inner goddess. Send a beam of light from your heart to her heart. See Aphrodite, the goddess of love, standing above the two of you with her hands on each of your heads, pouring divine love into you both. See this love circulating down from your heads to your hearts and then extending out to each others' hearts. In your imagination, speak gently to your friend from your heart. Ask her to speak gently to you from her heart, too.

Ask the Goddess to Bless Your Friendship

Put the entire situation into the Goddess's hands. Ask her to bring divine love and light to the situation. Ask her to speak through you the next time you see your friend. Ask her to bless your friendship and work through you and your friend so you can resolve things amicably.

Focus on What Is Working in Your Friendship

Think about all the things you love about your friend. So often when we are mad it is easy to get caught up in all the things that irritate you about her. Even if your whole friendship feels like a mess, think about some things that are good about the relationship.

When You Feel Centered Reach Out to Your Friend from Your Heart

When you feel like you can see the bigger picture, call your friend and ask if you can talk about things. Remember to keep praying, asking the Goddess to help you speak from your heart and not get caught up in personality issues. Ask the Goddess to speak through you. Tell your friend what you love and appreciate about her, and let her know that her friendship is important to you and you are willing to work through this stuff with her. Tell her that you guys are a team and that you can face this problem together, no matter how difficult it may seem. Be patient, persistent, and willing to listen with an open heart and open mind. Instead of blaming, try talking about how you feel, and if she gets into blaming you for stuff, try asking her how that makes her feel instead of reacting to the blame.

Trust the Future of Your Friendship

Very special friends will stick with you through thick and thin. They put up with all your idiosyncrasies just as you put up with theirs. That's what is so special about having a best friend. You know you can count on them, no matter what. But sometimes relationships change form and there may come a time when you no longer want her for a best friend or she no longer wants you for a best friend. Sometimes best friends can move away and that is very sad, too. When you are the one being dumped, it can be devastating. If this happens, ask the Goddess to encircle you with love and know that even though it may feel like the end of the world at the time, it's not. Trust me on this, okay! You will have many friends over the course of your lifetime, and what you shared with one person will always be special, even if the outer form changes.

Mahuika's Magical Breastplate

In the Celtic tradition a magical breastplate is called a lorica. Remember we talked about loricas in the chapter on Queen Boadicea. A lorica is a prayer you say to call on divine protection from different sources, such as the sun, the moon, the stars, your ancestors, God, the angels, and the Goddess. You use an incantation to weave the prayer around your body. An incantation is a spoken spell. As you say your lorica you imagine a beautiful breastplate forming around your torso to protect you from harm. A lorica can protect you from other people's negative energy. It can protect you from getting your heart hurt when you are around an ex-boyfriend who you still have feelings for. It protects you from people who send you angry or hateful glances or thoughts, or who say mean things about you, either to you or to others. Basically, a lorica protects you from any kind of harm.

There are many similarities between the Maoris and the Celts. They were both tribal people. They were both warrior races. They both believed the spirit was contained inside the head, and they would collect the heads of their enemies after they had killed them to increase their *mana* (spiritual power). They were both oral traditions and believed the spoken word was sacred—that you were saying spoken spells every time you talked. They both practiced magical tattooing, did hakas before entering into battle, and practiced a form of boasting before fighting to intimidate their enemies and invoke spiritual power.

These are just a few of the similarities. I find it interesting that so many people of Celtic descent traveled to New Zealand in the last couple hundred years and married Maori people or people of Maori descent. My grandmother was Maori and she married a Celtic man—my grandfather was from Ireland and of Celtic descent. My mother therefore had both Maori and Celtic blood. As do I—from her and from my dad, whose family descends from Scotland, another Celtic land. Joining the Celtic and Maori bloodlines makes potent magic, I believe. I often feel the presence of my warrior ancestors around me.

The Maoris dressed themselves spiritually and physically before battle. They did not wear physical breastplates but had their tattoos and their incantations to protect them from harm. Spiritual dressing was just as important to them as physical dress. They would not leave home without putting their spiritual clothes on, just like we wouldn't think of leaving home without our regular clothes. To do so for them would be to invite trouble. They would feel naked without their spiritual garments.

The most famous lorica is "The Breastplate of St. Patrick," also called "The Deer's Cry." I do not know the Maori word for a lorica, so if you are reading this and do know it, please send it to me!

Anyway, here is Mahuika's magical breastplate to invoke your own goddess power. As you say it, feel the power of each element radiating through you. Draw power up from the earth into your body and down from the sky and the mountains and the trees. Close your eyes after reading each line and imagine what you are saying. Visualize a beautiful breastplate weaving around your body.

I arm myself today with

The strength of the sun

The magnetism of the moon

The stability of the mountains

The fluidity of the oceans.

I arm myself today with

The knowledge of the rocks

The wisdom of the trees

The heartbeat of the earth.

I arm myself today with

The power of the Goddess

May her words be my words

Her sight be my sight

Her hearing be my hearing

Her knowledge be my knowledge

Her wisdom be my wisdom

Her truth be my truth

Her power be my power

Her strength be my strength

Her love be my love.

May the Goddess and my ancestors guard me today

From all who wish me harm

In thoughts, words, or deeds

Here and afar.

The Goddess above me and below me

The Goddess before me and behind me

The Goddess at my right and my left

The Goddess around me and about me

With me and within me

I arm myself with the power of the Goddess

And so it is

As you say the final verse, that is the time to really visualize a beautiful breast-plate weaving around you. You can also see angels and spiritual warriors standing around you, too, for extra protection. Plus you can use jewelry, perfume, and clothing to enhance your lorica, just like when you throw a glamour.

Mahuika's Glamour

- Blue lipstick

- Black eyeliner

- Temporary tattoos in spiral or tribal designs

- Create your own *moko*, or personal signature, which tells the story of your lineage—where you came from and what you want to achieve through your mother's family line

- Fiery red nail polish

Makeup

Have a shower and wash your hair. Blow-dry it gently or let it dry naturally. Mahuika was not one to fuss with elaborate hairdos. Keep your makeup simple, too. Use black eyeliner or dark green eyeliner to line your eyes. Apply a dark brown shadow to your eyelids and then line your eyes with the eyeliner, drawing a thick line from the inner corner of your eye across the lid to the outer corner. Then draw a line under your lower lashes as close to the lashes as possible.

Next use a green eyeliner to line your lips and a blue lipstick to fill them in. Remember, blue lips were a sign of great beauty in the Maori tradition. If you feel weird with blue lipstick just use a clear lip gloss. Many makeup companies make blue lipstick now, like L'Oreal and Hard Candy.

Draw your own moko either on your chin or on your arm using a tattoo pen (which you can buy at drugstores) or the dark green eyeliner. Use a symbol that is meaningful to you. Think of your moko as your logo. This is a drawing that represents you, your family, and your tribe. It says who you are.

Add some temporary tattoos in tribal or spiral designs and you are ready to go.

Clothing

Traditionally Maori women wore flax skirts with embroidered bodices and embroidered headbands. When I was in school one of our projects for social studies each year would be to embroider a Maori headband. You can wear a bandanna around your head instead or find a pretty headband. For the clothing, try a little top with spaghetti straps and a comfortable skirt or sarong. Red, white, and black are the colors that the Maori women wear today in their traditional dress.

Ceremony

I like *Oceania* by Oceania (Polygram Records, May 2000), which is Maori trance music, and *Shaman's Breath* by Professor Trance and the Energizers (Polygram Records, January 1995). Turn up the music loud. Close your eyes and call out to Mahuika:

Mahuika

Great goddess of fire, power, and strength

Bring your power to me now

Let it fill every pore of my being

Radiate from me your strength and brilliant glory

Fill me with your power

Fill me with your power

Fill me with your power

Keep chanting "Fill me with your power" until you really do feel as if you are filled with the magnificent power of Mahuika. Feel her confidence, certainty, and strength filling you and radiating from you.

Now see a band of warriors standing around you, facing outwards. These can be Maori warriors, Celtic warriors, or warriors from a tradition that you feel an affinity with. These warriors are strong and powerful. They are invincible. They stand in a warrior stance ready to attack anyone who wishes to harm you. They hold in their hands long, strong spears with the tips burning brightly with fire. They will not hesitate to use these flaming spears on anyone who threatens you.

You feel safe and protected by your warrior allies. You know you can call on them any time when you feel scared or vulnerable. You can call on them to help you before you go into battle or before a competition or if you are at home alone. You can call on them when you have a social event and you feel shy for protection and confidence or you can call on them when some guy or girl is hassling you.

You know, too, that you can call on them and imagine them surrounding your home when you go to bed at night or when you are gone for the day. Plus you can ask them to surround your loved ones and your belongings for protection. These are your very own spiritual bodyguards.

Mahuika's Tasks for You

- Dress as Mahuika for one day this week. How does it feel to be a fiery goddess of strength and power? Write about it in your goddess journal.

- Say a lorica each morning this week before you leave the house. Practice dressing yourself in magical garments as well as in physical clothes.

- Pay attention to the words you use. What kinds of sacred contracts are you creating with your words?

- Read *Celebrating the Southern Seasons* by Juliet Batten (Tandem Press, 1995) if you would like more information on Celtic and Maori ceremonies.

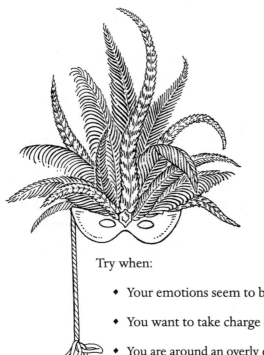

Oshun

....

**THE WATER
GODDESS**

Try when:

- ◆ Your emotions seem to be all over the place

- ◆ You want to take charge of your life

- ◆ You are around an overly emotional person
who drains you

Oshun (pronounced *oh-shun*, like ocean), who is sometimes known also as Erzulie, is the African goddess of love from the Yoruba tradition. Beauty, love, and sensuality are her creations. Her name means "of the mountains" and she is a water goddess. Water is very sacred in Africa because the climate is so dry. The Water Goddess rules the realm of emotions. She can calm turbulent waters and soothe raging storms.

One story was that Earth and Storm had an argument. Earth went underground in a fit of anger. Storm thought Earth had taken fire and water with her, so he could not provide rain for the people. The people suffered terribly without water. Eventually Storm realized that Earth had not taken fire and water away, so he created lightning and made the rain fall again.

Oshun heals with cooling waters. Any time you are by a river, lake, waterfall, or creek, you are in her magnificent presence. Listen softly for the sound of her soul singing upon the babbling of the waters. Oshun carries within herself the power of love. She gives substance and form to love and plants it firmly within Earth's steadying influence. One of her greatest qualities is her ability to ground emotions and give them a solid form in which to gestate and grow.

Oshun knows her true worth, therefore she is able to pick a partner worthy of her. She is full of self-confidence. She knows love is as endless and vast as the ocean—that you are a vessel for love and the bigger the container, the greater the amount of love you can receive. If you take a thimble to the ocean, then a thimbleful of water is all you will be able to carry home, and so it is with love. Oshun motions you to open your heart wide to the presence of love and to manifest it on solid ground.

Oshun's Story

How Oshun learned to read the sacred seashells

Once upon a time, a long, long time ago, there lived a beautiful goddess named Oshun. Oshun's skin was as brown as the richest, most decadent chocolate. Her ebony hair was a mass of ringlets. This goddess was gorgeous and when she applied honey to her pulse points, no one could resist her sweet allure.

Now Oshun desired to learn how to read the seashells, the sacred gifts from the ocean floor, which could foretell the future if you knew how to read them. There was only one other deity that could do this, and that was Obtala, the great deity. Obtala was neither man nor woman; s/he had qualities of both. He was as ancient as the oldest rocks upon the Earth and his face was as weathered as them, too! Obtala wore a gown of luminous white like the snow covering the mountains, which glistened in the sunlight and the moonlight.

Obtala was the kindest, wisest, and most powerful of all the Yoruba deities. He kept the peace with his wise counsel. And it was Obtala who shaped the babies in their mother's womb and who was deeply empathetic with mortals' concerns.

Oshun went to Obtala to ask him to teach her how to read the shells, but Obtala refused. So again Oshun went to Obtala and begged, "Please, Baba, please teach me how to read the sacred shells." But again Obtala refused her. This went on for several months and each time Oshun asked, Obtala was adamant in his refusal.

So Oshun, who was by this time getting quite frustrated, decided she had best change tactics. She decided to bide her time and learn how best she might approach Obtala and win his trust. She waited by the river until Obtala came down from his mountaintop home to bathe. She watched as Obtala let the luminous gown drop from his body onto the sandy shore and elegantly strode into the cool, refreshing water. And she saw Elegba, the trickster god, sneak out of the bushes and snatch up Obtala's gown and run away with it!

Oshun moved closer to the water and began picking flowers along the river's edge, humming to herself.

"Oh, good morning, Obtala!" she grinned as Obtala caught her eye.

"Why, good morning, Oshun," he replied. "Lovely to see you, you are looking radiant as ever!"

"Yes, indeed," she smiled. "I am feeling particularly fortunate this morning."

Before Obtala could ask Oshun what was the reason for her good fortune, he reached out to grab his gown and got a handful of sand in its place.

"My gown!" he roared.

Oshun frowned with fake concern. "Why, whatever is the matter, Obtala?" she queried.

"My clothes are gone! I left them here when I came in to bathe, and now my beautiful gown is missing. How can I be the King of White Cloth without my ceremonial clothes? Oshun, I will be a laughingstock."

Oshun cocked her head to the side for a moment and pretended to think.

"I tell you what, Obtala. If I find your gown for you, will you teach me to read the shells?"

Obtala looked at Oshun with a hint of suspicion darkening his craggy face. But he admired her shrewdness and he replied, "Well, Oshun, if you can find it, then yes," he relented. "I will teach you to read the shells."

Oshun ran home to change. She dressed in five yellow silk scarves tied around her waist. She sprayed honey all over her skin so that her body glistened and radiated the sweet perfume. She picked up her favorite fan and quickly made her way to Elegba's home.

"Elegba," she called out, knocking on the door. "Elegba! You must give me Obtala's gown."

Elegba bounded down the stairs to his front door and nearly knocked Oshun over. He glanced up at her.

"Wow, Oshun," he enthused. "You look great!"

270

"That may be, Elegba," smiled Oshun coquettishly, for she knew her true worth. "But what I really want is for you to give me back Obtala's clothes."

But all Elegba could think about was kissing Oshun and how wonderful that would feel. So they came to a compromise, where Elegba got his kisses and Oshun got the gown, and they were both satisfied—for Oshun was quite a bit attracted to Elegba, too.

Then Oshun made her way back to the river and gave Obtala his gown, and in return he taught her how to hold the shells and listen to them and divine the future and the past. And he taught her how to shake them and cast them upon the sand and interpret their meanings from the way they landed.

After she had practiced the secret of the shells, she gathered together the other Orishas (gods) and taught them how to use the shells, too.

Magic in Africa

Magic is considered very powerful in Africa, even today. People use talismans and gris-gris (amulets) to protect themselves from injury, disease, illness, wounds, enemies, and even from thieves! Amulets are used to bring the wearer wealth and good fortune.

African religion teaches that the world and everything in it must be obedient to the shaman or medicine man (magician). The magicians have the power to command the elements. People believe the soul lives on after death. So magicians call on the power of their ancestors and other souls to aid their powers.

The souls of the dead can reincarnate into animals or plants as well as to human beings. The Zulus won't kill certain types of snakes if they think the snake contains the spirit of their relative.

Africans believe all objects, animate and inanimate, have a spirit. These spirits come from a particular deity. There are two types of spirits: the spirits of natural phenomena like rivers, plants, trees, and rocks, and the spirits of the ancestors.

Each family has special ceremonies and sacred stories for their ancestors. The ancestors often take on legendary proportions after death and gain a demigod status.

Sickness and death are not attributed to natural causes. Instead, they are seen as vengeance caused by evil spirits.

Medicine men are greatly respected within the tribe. They hold positions of high authority. They practice as specialists in many different areas. For example, a person who is going on a hunt will go see a medicine man first to get an amulet for successful hunting. There are medicine men for everything from whirlwinds to alligators and panthers to pregnant women! If someone is the victim of a crime, they can consult a medicine man who specializes in discerning who the criminal was.

Some medicine men specialize in making rain. They perform sacred ceremonies where they hold a gourd containing seeds that have been blessed and shake it with their right hand, chanting invocations to produce rain.

During the ceremony, the medicine man puts on a special costume and mask to represent the deity he wishes to invoke. Using dance and music—often drumming—the shaman becomes the deity he or she is invoking, which gives him or her the special powers, like healing or manifesting, of the deity, just like you can do when you throw a glamour.

Santería and Yoruba are two religions from Africa that are also practiced in the United States. The Voodoo religion of Haiti comes partly from the different religions and traditions of African slaves. The deities and spirits are divided into two groups: helpful "rada" and trouble-making "petro" spirits (from *The Larousse Encyclopedia of Mythology*).

The Water Goddess

Many love goddesses come from the sea. Water is often a symbol of emotions and love in mythology, tarot, and dream interpretations. The Water Goddess is a great goddess to go to when you want more love in your life. She contains an endless supply of nourishment to sustain our lives. Without physical, emotional, mental, and spiritual juice our lives become dry and destitute, and we rot away.

The Water Goddess can teach you the nature of your feelings. She will show you how to control the ebb and flow of your moods and desires. She helps you to integrate your emotions after a period of soul-searching or loss.

In mythology, water often represents our emotions and, indeed, our emotions are often pulled by many tides around us. Water magic is great for purifying and cleansing, and for getting in touch with the flow of our creativity and our magic.

Water People

Physically, water people have large, expressive eyes. They often have a far-off look in them, too, with a dreamy expression, as if they are looking off across the ocean to far-off shores. They have curvaceous, flowing bodies with soft, moist skin. Emotionally they make changes almost constantly. They can be like a joyful, bubbling brook one moment and like a turbulent tidal wave the next! Water people are very intuitive, dreamy, and creative. They use their powers of insight and reflection to give them a deeper perception of life and people around them.

Keeping Water In Balance

Just the right amount of water in your being gives you a great amount of creativity and the ability to act on your ideas. You have great dreams and work to manifest them. You are loving and in tune with your emotions without being overemotional.

Too Little Water

Too little water in your being leads to blocked creativity and trouble identifying feelings. Someone who has a lack of water finds it difficult to express their feelings and to relate to others. They are not very empathetic. These people try too hard to be self-sufficient and don't like to be dependent on anyone else. They hate asking for help.

Too Much Water

If you have too much water, try:

* Eating earth foods to soak up some of that water, like bread, potatoes, and pasta

* Doing some form of strength training—try fifteen minutes of free weights or calisthenics every day to give you more definition, physically and emotionally

* Building up your mental fitness—you must learn how to manage your moods and condition yourself emotionally (follow the guidelines in this chapter)

How to Get More Water

If you think you may need more water, try:

* Wearing shimmery blue clothes

* Eating seafood

* Drinking lots of water

* Going for a swim

* Wearing jewelry from the sea like pearls, shells, coral, opals, or abalone

What If You Have Too Much Water?

Too much water will make you overemotional. You will find it difficult to make a decision and will often change your mood or your mind, depending on who you are hanging out with. You have trouble managing your moods and emotions and may often find yourself depressed or melancholic without knowing how to snap out of it. People who have a lot of water are most prone to suicidal thoughts

273

simply because they don't know how to turn things around. Water people are sensitive to their environment and can let external circumstances wash them around. They can be clingy and insecure. They may be highly creative and come up with great ideas but have trouble taking action.

Playing Weather Goddess

How to direct your moods and others' moods

Like the African shamans who direct the outside weather, you can learn to direct the weather of your emotions and of those around you. Managing your moods is the most empowering skill you can learn as part of your goddess training. Some people never learn how to manage their moods. They go through life letting circumstances dictate to them how they should feel. They can feel overwhelmed by their emotions and unwittingly stay stuck in painful emotions without learning how to move forward. Kurt Cobain is a good example of someone famous who never learned how to manage his moods. He had things most people only dream about—fame, fortune, a beautiful wife and daughter. But because he didn't know how to manage his bad feelings, he chose drugs as a way of medicating himself, and eventually he chose death.

When you learn how to manage your moods, you realize you always have a choice. Bad stuff may happen but you know you can deal with it. You may feel lousy from time to time but you take deliberate action to get out of the pain as quickly as possible. A bad thought or painful memory may pop into your mind but you don't invite it to hang out with you and ruin the rest of your life!

Oshun is the mistress of managing her moods. There's no way she lets other people or outer circumstances determine how she feels! She knows she is in charge of her life. As I have said repeatedly throughout this book, sometimes you don't have a whole lot of control over what happens to you, but you *always* have control over how you respond.

Think of yourself as a weather goddess as you practice mood management. Just like the African shamans, there are certain actions you can take to invoke different moods. Some days storms will roll in, the winds will blow and rain may pelt down—however, you have the inner power to withstand even the wickedest weather. Not only can you withstand it but you can turn it around so you can gain something from it.

Once you know how to manage your moods, then you can learn how to manage other people's, too. The point of learning how to manage others' moods is not to manipulate them to do what you want but to prevent sticky situations from escalating. Emotional maturity requires you learn how to stop reacting to others and stay centered and focused on a productive outcome.

Managing Your Moods

There are two main ways to manage your moods:

1. Change your physiology (move your body)

2. Change your mental focus (this is divided into two parts, changing *what* you focus on or changing *how* you focus on it)

Change Your Physiology

When you have a day when you feel depressed or you feel angry, do something physical about it. Your body movement has an enormous impact on the way you feel emotionally.

....
Goddess Workout

Close your eyes for a moment and think about someone who is depressed. How do they stand? Everything is facing downwards, right? Their head is down, their shoulders are crunched down, their eyes are downcast, their lips are down, the volume of their voice is down, their energy is down. Take a moment to stand like this. It is pretty hard to feel "up" when your body is in this state.

Now throw your shoulders back, hold your tummy in, breathe deeply, put your head up high, and plaster a big silly grin on your face. Just by doing this simple move, you are increasing your energy and changing your emotional state.

Think of some moves you can make when you feel crappy to get your body into a more empowered stance. Jumping jacks are good, as is standing tall, going for a brisk walk, stretching your body, or shaking your head vigorously from side to side. Speak strongly, deepen your voice, and speak with passion. Use emotive language; say things like "I'm fantastic!" when people ask how you are. Look up powerful words in a thesaurus that you can use to describe your emotions. Try saying words like *brilliant, wonderful, jazzed*, and phrases like "I'm great and getting better!" Pretend you are Steve Irwin, the crocodile hunter, and practice using his intonations to deliver your words.

People who do yoga or tai chi know that breathing can immediately change your emotions. Take ten deep breaths and close your eyes the next time you feel stressed out.

Change Your Mental Focus

This step is divided into two parts. When an upsetting thought or feeling comes along, toss it out and think about something else or change the way you think about it.

Our minds are constantly making mental pictures. Our minds are very much like video cameras. Every situation we are in, our mind focuses on different happenings just like a video camera does. We zoom in on different things and make them larger in our imagination. You may go to a party with your best friend and have two totally different experiences, depending on what each of you are focusing on.

Our memories are like video stores. Inside we have literally thousands of videos, or stored memories, which we can choose to play over and over. At times it is the sad, melancholic dramas from our lives that we replay on our mental movie screen, or the horror movie memories. The problem with this is when we replay painful events from our past, our body experiences the same feelings as when it first happened, so we are not in a very empowered state to act effectively. In my experience the more you relive a painful experience, the more likely you are to stay stuck.

What you need to do when that video comes on in your mind is press the "eject" button and put a different video in—put on a comedy or a happy ending. Hey, it is your mind—you can do what you like!

What if you are having a hard time thinking of something different? That old bad thought comes along and you try and try but you just can't seem to replace it with a different happy one. Well, you can take something that has caused you a lot of pain in the past and use your magic to make it smaller and lose its power. You can make it dissolve so it disappears completely.

How do you do this? Just like a movie director does! Movie directors work constantly to produce a certain emotion from their audience. They use music, color, graphics, camera angle, voice, posture, and tonality to create the response they want their viewers to experience. Movie directors know they can change the effect their movie has on an audience. In the same way, you can change the effect your mental movies have on you.

So the next time you find yourself viewing an old painful experience, do what a movie director does. Change the focus. Zoom out instead of doing a close-up, turn the volume down so you can't hear the voices so loudly, turn it into a cartoon, scramble up the images, give people who are being mean to you moustaches or hairy armpits. Turn their skin green, see them with huge red pimples all over their bodies. See the tape being all scratched up so you can't view it properly. Do whatever it takes to produce a different feeling.

I know this sounds simplistic. It is. But it works! These simple techniques have worked miracles in my life for lifting me out of crappy feelings. So try it and see for yourself—but remember, just like anything else, you have to practice.

Mental and emotional fitness are just the same as physical fitness. You can't work out once and expect to be fit the next day! You have to train every single day to get into peak condition. One of the most effective ways I have found to increase my mental and emotional fitness is to listen to a motivational tape every day. Use the same one over and over for thirty days. I like tapes by Anthony Robbins—see if you can borrow one from your local library. Don't forget to ask Oshun to help you with this.

Managing Others' Moods

It is quite easy to learn how to manage other people's moods. You just have to practice a few simple tricks. When you are around someone who is throwing a barney (tantrum) or doing something that makes you feel lousy, you don't have to just stand there and be exposed to it. You can walk out of the room, change the subject, or do something unexpected. Just because someone is saying garbage doesn't mean you have to ingest it.

I first learned how to do this with my dad. I love my dad. Sometimes he starts talking about stuff I did (or didn't do) when I was a teenager. This was years ago but he still manages to make me feel lousy about it! So whenever I'm around him and he starts in on one of those topics, I immediately change the subject. I say something like: "Remember when . . ." and start talking about something fun we did together. He forgets what he was talking about and we have a great conversation. Or I ask him a question about something interesting that he is good at.

The other thing my dad has a tendency to do is to be cantankerous. He can get grumpy for no apparent reason in a matter of seconds. I used to get cantankerous back and pretty soon we would be having a smashing argument. This wasn't very productive. Now when he is in one of those moods I just drift off into another room. I do this when I am around people who are having "pity parties" or talking a lot of gloom and doom. No point making yourself feel miserable by hanging around all that stuff.

But what if you are in a situation where you can't get away? Then use the movie director technique and tune them out mentally. Turn the volume down in your mind or think about something else. If you are in a situation where someone is abusive to you, report him or her. There are laws to deal with abuse.

··

Goddess Workout

Who is someone that you often feel miserable around when you hang out
with them?

What is it that they do or say that makes you feel miserable (or uptight)?

What three things could you do when they start in on their stuff?

1.

2.

3.

Practice this the next time you are with them.

Oshun's Beauty Ceremony to Start the Day

Another way to manage your moods is to know your true worth, and to remember you have the power to direct the focus of your day. You can set the energetic
tone for the day by focusing on what qualities you would like to radiate. Oshun is
the intoxicating goddess of beauty. She knows her true worth. Other people are
enchanted and mesmerized by her beauty. Call on her to increase your beauty. Let
her essence radiate through you so you become intoxicating, too.

1. Have a shower.

2. Sprinkle a few drops of essential oils on your skin. You can use ylang-ylang to radiate sexual confidence, lemon to pep you up, rosemary to increase your memory, lavender to soothe and comfort you, jasmine for allure, or sandalwood to enchant.

3. Wash your face with a gentle cleanser. Please don't use soap, even if it is special skin soap. Soap strips the skin of its acid/alkaline balance and dries it out.

4. Pat your skin dry, wrap your hair in a towel so it is off your face, and lather your face with moisturizer.

5. Apply sunscreen to your face.

6. Put your makeup on the bathroom counter.

7. Look into the mirror, gaze into your eyes, and think about Oshun and how beautiful she is, how confident she is, how sexy she is.

8. Pray: "O Great Goddess, whose name is famous through all of time, I do ask thee to assist me to conjure up a vision of thy beauty and thy strength for this day."

9. Let Oshun guide you to apply your makeup, clothing, and perfume to create a perfect look of beauty for today.

10. Apply a small amount of honey to your pulse points in Oshun's honor.

Oshun's Honey Body Lotion

Honey is an ancient beauty aid filled with vitamins and minerals. It is an excellent moisturizer and healer of skin. Use it liberally but beware—it is sticky!

You can make your own honey facial mask simply by applying honey all over your face after you have washed it. Leave on for twenty minutes, then rinse off with warm water and apply a light moisturizer.

Here is a recipe for a body lotion sacred to Oshun using honey, oranges, and cinnamon, which are all holy to her.

Mix four ounces sweet almond oil with two ounces honey, one tablespoon orange juice, three tablespoons of water, and a pinch of cinnamon or allspice. Put into a clean plastic bottle. Place your hands on the bottle and say a prayer to Oshun, asking her to bless the sacred lotion. Heat in the microwave for twenty seconds, then gently shake before applying to your skin (check temperature on the back of your hand first to ensure it is not hot). Do this facial in your bathrobe with your hair wrapped in a towel as it is sticky and may stick to your clothes.

Oshun's Glamour

- Yellow silk anything

- A beautiful yellow rose

- A fan

- Honey on the skin

- Rosy red cheeks

- Coral jewelry

- Shells and beads

- Perfume (something spicy, like Opium)

Makeup

Line your eyes with navy blue eyeliner and apply a creamy yellow shadow to your eyelids. Use a plain gloss on your lips and a light peach blush on your cheeks. Highlight your skin with gold glitter splashed across your collarbone.

Clothing

Wear a dress in any shade of yellow. Oshun loves yellow. Even though she is a water goddess and most water goddesses would wear blue—not Oshun. Wear shell earrings or a beautiful beaded necklace. You can make one yourself, praying to Oshun while you make it. Carry a fan—Oshun *loves* fans.

Ceremony

Make an altar for Oshun. Remember, she loves beauty so make it as beautiful as you can. Place a yellow candle, a shell, a fan, a small jar of honey and five pumpkin seeds on the altar as offerings to Oshun.

Close your eyes and say a prayer to Oshun:

Dearest Oshun

Goddess of beauty, water, and power

I ask thee to fill me

With your power, beauty, and confidence

Descend upon me now

You can ask Oshun for something you desire, too. She is great for bringing you boyfriends, increasing your beauty, giving you confidence, or teaching you how to manage your moods.

Feel her power, strength, and confidence radiate through you. Do something you have been procrastinating over and ask for her help.

If there is an emotion or memory you have been having a hard time with, get five pennies and hold them, thinking about what it is you wish to be free of. Ask Oshun to heal the emotion. Take the pennies to the nearest river or body of water and throw them in, releasing the situation completely to Oshun.

Oshun's Tasks for You

- Spend a day as Oshun. How does it feel to be a goddess of water who is totally in control of her moods? Write about your experience in your goddess journal.

- Choose one person who has been bugging you and change the way you act when you are around them. How do you feel when you take action to control your emotions?

- Choose a memory that has been haunting you. Try the "director" technique and smoosh it up in your imagination. Turn it into a cartoon. Add silly graphics. Keep practicing until the memory loses its power over you.

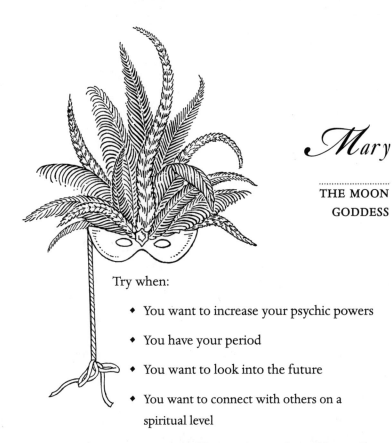

Mary

....

THE MOON
GODDESS

Try when:

- You want to increase your psychic powers

- You have your period

- You want to look into the future

- You want to connect with others on a
  spiritual level

Mary is a moon goddess and a triple goddess. She is often
shown with a halo around her head that looks like a full
moon encircled with stars. Sometimes she is pictured standing
on a crescent moon like the high priestess in traditional tarot
decks. The gifts of the moon goddess are psychic messages
(especially with clairvoyance) and the ability to see things
from the spirit realm, such as angels and visions for the future.
In Mary's story, you will see how she does that.

Mary is often seen as an intercessor between people and
the God triune in the Christian tradition. People pray to her
to pass on their requests to God, Jesus, or the Holy Spirit.

Sometimes people seek the advice of clairvoyants or psy-
chics to receive spiritual information. In the goddess tradition,

you can talk directly to God or Goddess. Three is a sacred number in many spiritual traditions, including the goddess tradition.

Mary's Story

Maiden, mother, and crone, the three faces of the moon

Mary the Maiden

Once upon a time, a long, long time ago, there lived a beautiful young woman named Mary in the city of Nazareth in the south part of Galilee. Galilee was a Roman province between the Mediterranean Sea and the Jordan River. Mary was happily engaged to a kind man named Joseph. He loved her for her sweetness and her compassion and the way he felt whenever he was around her.

In those days engagements lasted for an entire year and it was very important that the betrothed did not have sex during that time because their laws forbade sex before marriage.

One day a beautiful angel with long brown hair and shining blue eyes came to visit Mary. This was Gabriel, the archangel of communication. "Mary," she said, "rejoice, for you are highly favored. The Lord is with you and you are blessed among women."

Gabriel continued. "And what is more, you will conceive the Son of God in your womb and his name will be Jesus, and he will be known as the son of the highest. God will give him the throne of his father David, and he will reign over the house of Jacob forever."

"How can this be?" Mary questioned. "I am still a virgin. I have never had sex with Joseph. Indeed, if I did before we are married, I could be stoned to death for my crime."

"The Holy Spirit will come upon you, Mary," answered Gabriel. "Do not be afraid, for you have found favor with God and his power will protect you."

After Gabriel had left, Mary went to visit her relative Elizabeth. She knocked on the door, then entered, calling out "hello" to Elizabeth. When Elizabeth heard Mary, she was filled with the Holy Spirit and began to pray: "Blessed are you

284

among women and blessed is the fruit of your womb." She did this even though she had no idea previously that Mary was pregnant.

Next Mary went to tell Joseph about the events of the day and how she was now pregnant. Joseph was alarmed at first. He knew Mary would be stoned and killed once people found out she was pregnant. He was tortured about what to do, for he didn't want any harm to come to Mary. Maybe it would be best if Mary were hidden away until after the baby was born, he thought.

That night he tossed and turned during his sleep, all these worries racing through his mind. Suddenly a brilliant angel appeared in his dreams. "Joseph," he said, "do not be afraid, for the baby conceived in Mary is of the Holy Spirit. Take her as your wife and have no fear of her being harmed."

So when Joseph awoke, he did as the angel said and married Mary. Not too much later, the baby Jesus was born.

Mary the Mother

Every year Mary and Joseph went with a group of friends and family to Jerusalem to the Feast of Passover. When Jesus was twelve they took him, too. After the feast Mary and Joseph headed back home, thinking Jesus was among them all. However, Jesus had decided to stay behind without telling anyone. They had been traveling for a day when they realized he was missing. Frantically they searched for him, and finally decided to return to Jerusalem to see if he was there.

Three worried days later, they found him in a temple talking with the teachers there. The teachers were amazed at his wisdom. So were his parents, but Mary gently reprimanded him: "Son, why have you done this to us? Your father and I have been worried sick looking for you." And Jesus replied, "You did not need to seek me, for you know I must be about my Father's business."

And Mary realized in that moment that Jesus was no longer a child, and that it was time for her to let him make his own decisions about his life.

Mary the Crone

On the day of Jesus' execution, Mary's heart was filled with grief. So deep was her sense of loss, she had never felt pain this intense as she walked to the place where

Jesus would die. Looking at her son with love, Mary knew this was the last time she would ever hear his voice, touch his face, or feel his heart beating on this earthly plane. This was the son she had borne from her own body, flesh from flesh, life from life, begotten not made.

She remembered the first time she had held him in her arms and seen his tiny face all scrunched up and crying. She remembered the bittersweet pain of finding out she was pregnant, wondering how she would cope and whether she would be outcast or killed for her situation, pregnant before marriage. She remembered how scared she had felt then and how she had walked through her challenges with faith and how it had all been okay in the end.

And she felt scared now, looking at her dear son, her eldest son, the first baby to make her a mother, wondering again how she could possibly live through this. "O God," she wept silently, "how could you do this to me? If there is any way possible, please don't take him from me." For she knew in her heart that he was innocent of the charges made upon him.

Then she watched as her son's hands were held on the cross and huge nails were hammered into his wrists into the wood, and she watched as the blood spurted from the wounds. And she watched as her son's feet were held on the cross and huge nails were hammered into his flesh, into the wood. And she felt her body convulse. She felt the bile rising in her stomach and she turned and threw up on the ground behind her. And she screamed in agony, falling faint to the ground, tears flowing desperately from her eyes. There were no words to describe this pain. It filled every cell of her body, relentlessly. Her friends grabbed her arms, as if the strength of their lifeblood could pulse into her body and support her, too.

The next few days were a haze. Crucifixion was not a quick way to die. Mary didn't know if Jesus had died from lack of blood or from suffocation, when he was so tired he could no longer lift his head to breathe. Looking back, Mary couldn't remember how she made it through. On the third day after Jesus' crucifixion Mary walked with Mary Magdalene to the tomb were Jesus' body lay. They carried spices and oils so they could anoint his body. It was early in the morning and the women watched the sun rise above the horizon and paint yellow and red splashes across the lightening sky. As they walked, they asked each other, "Who will roll away the stone from the front of the tomb? It is so large. Surely it will be too heavy for us."

But when they arrived at the tomb, they saw that the stone had already been rolled away. Curious, they entered the tomb and saw that Jesus' body was gone. Suddenly two angels appeared, their robes shining brilliantly, and they smiled at the women. One of the angels said, "Why do you seek the living among the dead? He is not here. He has risen! Remember how he told you he would be crucified and would rise again on the third day."

And the women remembered how Jesus had foretold these events, and they quickly went to spread the word to the others.

Mary was human and, like every human, was capable of feeling inconsolable grief and sorrow. From an earthly perspective Mary felt the cruelty and injustice of losing her son. However, Mary also believed in God's divine will for her life. She knew from a spiritual perspective that Jesus had a divine mission to fulfill on Earth, just as she did.

In order to be able to witness the miracle of Jesus' resurrection, Mary first had to walk through dark moments of unbearable despair during his death. Her faith was tested but her trust in God and her belief in divine love was strengthened. Her pain was a portal into deeper empathy and compassion with the human spirit.

About Mary

Although Mary is not officially a goddess in the Christian tradition, she meets the goddess criteria according to the dictionary. As I said in the first chapter, one of the dictionary definitions of a goddess is a greatly adored woman. Mary is certainly one of the most beloved figures in Western religion. Early Christianity was opposed to the worship of goddesses. However, one of the earliest churches was on the site of the temple of the goddess Diana at Ephesus and dedicated to Mary (Pennick and Jones, *A History of Pagan Europe*, p. 75). In 431 a synod held at Ephesus first declared Mary as the mother of God. In the processional ceremony celebrating the blessedness of Mary, smoking censors containing incense were used and flaring torches were held, just like in the processions dedicated to Diana, who is also a moon goddess. Mary lived in a house near Ephesus at the end of her life, too.

There is evidence that there were religious groups dedicated to Mary, where she was worshipped in similar ways to the earlier Pagan goddesses.

People pray to Mary every day. If you want to talk to her, just see her in your imagination and begin a conversation with her, or you can use one of her prayers. You can light a candle before you begin to create sacred space, or you can light a candle when you ask her for your request.

Mary's Prayers

The Song of Mary

My soul magnifies the Lord

My spirit rejoices in God my savior

For he has regarded the holy state of his maidservant

From now, many generations will call me blessed

For he who is mighty has done great things for me

And holy is his name

—Luke, Chapter 1, *Extreem Teen Bible*
(Thomas Nelson Publishers, 1999)

Novena to the Miraculous Mother Mary

O miraculous mother

With inspired confidence I call upon thee

To extend thy merciful loving kindness

So that thy powers of perpetual help

Will protect me

And assist me in my needs and difficulties

Please grant me my desire

(make your requests here)

And so mote it be

Amen

—Prayer adapted from a seven-day candle
(Reed Candle Co.)

Prayer to the Miraculous Virgin Mary

Hail Mary

Full of grace

The Lord is with thee

Blessed art thou among women

And blessed is the fruit of thy womb, Jesus

Holy Mary, Mother of God

Pray for us now and at the hour of our death

Amen

—Prayer from a seven-day candle
(Reed Candle Co.)

The Many Sacred Threes in the Goddess Tradition

Three phases of the moon: Waxing; full; waning

Three phases of female power: Maiden; Mother; Crone / Enchantress

Three gifts of female power: To give birth; to give life; to give death

Three phases of initiation for women: Menstruation; pregnancy; menopause

Three levels of initiation in the Goddess tradition: Novice, learning level; Priestess, teaching level; High Priestess, leadership level (In some traditions called Priestess, High Priestess, Witch Queen [must start three covens to be awarded this title—there's that three again!])

Three aspects of the Goddess in Celtic tradition: Maiden; Mother or Summer Queen; Crone/Enchantress or Lady of the Lake

Three phases of menstruation: New egg begins to mature; ovulation; menstruation

The Three Powers of Women

Mary is a triple goddess. This means she carries the wisdom of maiden, mother, and crone within her. In some cultures triple goddesses are divided into three single, different goddesses; in Greece, Artemis is the maiden, Selene is the mother, and Hecate is the crone. They also represent the three phases of the moon—maiden is the waxing moon, mother is the full moon, and crone is the waning moon.

In the Bible there are also three Marys: Mary, the mother of Jesus; Mary Magdalene; and Mary of Bethany. You can see this as another manifestation of the triple goddess, just as in the story of Bridget, where she is a triple goddess but there are also stories of three different Bridgets, which could be seen as one woman divided into three. Each one carries a different aspect of the Goddess.

In the Celtic tradition, the Morrigan is the goddess who has the ability to give birth, life, and death. She is the goddess of fertility and can help women conceive. She is the goddess of life and can bring mortally wounded warriors back from the brink of death. And she is the goddess of death and can bring death.

All women, like Mary, carry within them three powers. These are the power to give birth, the power to give life, and the power to give death.

Each transition that a woman makes, from maiden to mother to crone, is a doorway into initiation. Many magical traditions have three levels of initiation to attain mastery. In the Goddess tradition, in the first level you are a novice; the second, a priestess; and the third, a high priestess (these differ depending on the tradition). To pass each level you must undergo a certain amount of training and then an initiation ceremony.

In Dolores Ashcroft-Nowicki's book *The Tree of Ecstasy*, Dolores goes into great detail about the triple powers of women. I recommend you read her book for more information (see Further Reading at the back of this book).

The Power to Give Birth

Women have the power to give birth not just on a physical level but also on a spiritual level. A prospering woman is continuously giving birth—to her ideas, her dreams, and her visions. In occult circles women are well regarded for their ability to contact the spiritual realms. Women are naturally receptive in their psychic abilities—that's why the phrase "women's intuition" is so familiar. Women have also served as muses for many a man. That's where the phrase "behind every successful man is a powerful woman" comes from. History is filled with stories of creative men who were inspired by the women in their lives, whether they were a sister, lover, friend, mother, or wife. Women not only birth their own ideas and creativity, but they act as midwives to others' creativity, helping to bring it into the world.

Have you ever had the experience of seeing the potential in someone else and helping them to connect with it and use it in a productive way? Women do this through conversations, sharing ideas, or seeing a vision of the person in their full potential and relaying what they see so the other person is inspired to take action. Women often help others to take action, too. Sometimes women see the best in someone who appears to be wasting their talents, and help them to birth a new way of being in the world.

The Power to Give Life

Women are naturally more resilient than men. Girl babies are hardier than boy babies. Women live longer than men statistically, and there are more women in the world than men. Plus women have an amazing ability to adapt to their surroundings. Many immigrant families have settled in harsh, unfamiliar territories. Often it is the woman who holds the family together and sets up the hearth, the heart center of the household, to provide nurturance and stability for the others.

Physically a woman can feed a baby from her body, too. It is such an amazing feeling to know that you are responsible for keeping a baby alive through the milk that your body produces.

There also comes a time in every mother's life when she knows she must "cut the apron strings" and allow her child to make their own decisions, even if this means watching them make mistakes. This is what Mary underwent at the temple in Jerusalem when she found Jesus.

The Power to Give Death

All women who give birth also give death, for whomever is born must eventually die. Even labor carries a risk, although in Western countries this likelihood is decreased by modern medicine and technology. There is still a small percentage of women who die giving birth in the Western world today.

In past times and still in third world countries, women enter pregnancy knowing they may not live through the birth of their child. It is a journey made with courage and with love in order to bring another life into the world. Women have the tenacity of spirit to face this journey into the unknown, plus they have the faith to bring children into the world not knowing what the future will hold for them, either.

Mothers have also faced the formidable task of being willing to sacrifice their lives for the love of their children, both literally and at a soul level. Mothers will battle for their children, sometimes putting their own life on the line. There have been stories of mothers who risked their lives to save their child's. Many mothers also make the choice to sacrifice their own dreams and desires for a while to raise a family.

Some mothers, like Mary, have had the unbearable task of watching a child die. Women see their children going off to war not knowing if they will return, being mortally injured, kidnapped, or suffering from a terminal illness. The power to survive these incidents is amazing and surely divinely gifted.

Gifts of the Moon Goddess

There are many moon goddesses in many different cultures. Nearly every culture has a moon goddess like the Lady of the Lake, the moon goddess from Arthurian legend, or Marama, the Maori moon goddess, or Selene, the Greek moon goddess.

For a long time the magical, mystical nature of the moon has been admired by people all over the world.

When I first started writing this chapter I was not going to use a specific goddess. I wanted you to become attuned with the magic of the Moon Goddess herself. But then Mary kept tugging at me. She wanted to be in this book!

We are pulled by the moon both psychically and physically, just like Mary was pulling at me. When we feel a yearning to explore our psychic potential it is the Moon Goddess calling us. Physically the moon pulls us: our bodies are 90 percent water and the sea, which is a much bigger body of water than our little bodies, is pulled by the magnetic powers of the moon as well. Our menstrual cycle is often attuned with the moon, and our emotions can be affected by her, too.

293

The Moon Goddess will teach you about the power of your menstrual cycle, which waxes, wanes, and is full, just like the cycle of the moon. She will teach you the art of divination, so you can look into the future and envision the outcome of situations. She will teach you how to shine light on the invisible parts of life, to sense others' energy, and to enchant and allure others. Her power is immense and incredible. Meditate on her face for twenty minutes each night for one month. You will find yourself becoming more magnetic, more psychic, and more magical. Try it and see.

There are three cards in the tarot that relate to the moon goddess. One is the High Priestess, who is a moon goddess. When you get this card in a reading it means it is time for you to focus on your spiritual path. It can also mean you will receive divine guidance or a spiritual teacher will be showing up in your life.

The other cards are the Star card and the Moon card. Both have water in them, showing the connection between the celestial realms and the ocean.

Menstrual Magic

Just as the moon has three stages in her cycle each month, moving from new to full to waning/dark, so, too, do you. The following is based on a typical twenty-eight-day cycle. Your cycle may not be exactly twenty-eight days—some girls' cycles are slightly longer, some shorter—but the process is the same.

Your Menstrual Cycle

DAYS 1–5

This is when you have your period. Your uterus is shedding its lining at the same time a new group of ova are forming in your ovaries.

DAYS 6–13

Your waxing moon time starts the day after you stop bleeding. The ova begins to mature into an ovum within your ovaries. The lining in your uterus (womb) is becoming thick and rich with nutrients in case of a possible pregnancy.

During your waxing moon time, you may find lots of new ideas, inspiration, and images come to you. Make the most of this time by beginning new projects, making notes in your goddess journal of your ideas, and drawing pictures or writing poems. Your energy and confidence is likely to be increased, too, so use this time wisely to tackle projects. Work prolifically and plan social events, go out with friends and have fun—this is a good time to be active.

DAY 14

Ovulation occurs, about fourteen days after the first day of your period. By now your uterine lining is twice as thick as it was at the end of your period on day five.

DAYS 14–19

The follicle that has the maturing egg inside it disintegrates, enabling the egg to move out toward the womb. This journey takes about five to six days and your released egg is transported by peristaltic contractions of the fallopian tube. You may notice your cervical mucus is clear and fluid and you might have a slight discharge. This looks like a small sticky spot in your underpants.

During ovulation you are fertile—you are in your full moon phase. Your personal magnetism is high, just like the full moon in the night sky. You can use your moon power to enchant or seduce others with great success. This is a perfect time for attracting a new boyfriend, getting a new job, or drawing your heart's desires to you. Use this time for manifesting what you most desire. You may find your glamours are especially strong at this time.

DAYS 20–28

The ovum reaches your uterus. If pregnancy did not occur, the ovum has dissolved—usually by day twenty.

Beginning on day twenty-one, the lining of your uterus starts to deteriorate. This breaking down of the lining continues until day twenty-eight. Then the uterus begins to shed the blood and the watery tissues of the lining.

DAYS 1–5

Now we are back to when the uterine lining is being shed and you are having your period.

The time just before your period and while you are bleeding is your waning moon time. This is when you enter the wise woman phase. Now more than ever you have access to all your psychic abilities. This is an excellent time to perform banishings of any kind, to channel the Goddess, and to do psychic work or astral travel. Use this time to test your clairvoyant powers and to have regular conversations with the angels and the goddesses. Your energy may be low during your waning moon time, so use it wisely. Stay home and write in your journal, take catnaps, and practice your magic instead of participating in vigorous social activities. If you like, you can save some of your menstrual blood to use in spells. Your menstrual blood is packed with nutrients and powerful energy. You can use a smudge on candles. This blood would have sustained life if you had become pregnant during ovulation.

In olden times, women were seen as unclean when they were menstruating. The Bible has lots of references to "unclean" women who were menstruating. In those days, women had to sacrifice birds as penance for being unclean. The ancient Romans thought menstrual blood was deadly and could make a dog's bite poisonous if the dog had tasted menstrual blood!

In reality, women are at their most potent psychically when they are menstruating. So use your psychic powers consciously.

······························

Goddess Workout

Make your own lunar calendar to mark your menstrual cycle.

Get a regular calendar. Begin marking the first day of your new moon time on the first day after you next stop bleeding. Each evening write a few lines about how you felt, your emotions, any food cravings you noticed, how your body felt, and your energy level. After three months you will know your own cycle pretty well and will be able to use it to predict when you are at your most creative and energetic and when you need to take it easy.

By charting your monthly cycle you will tune into your powerful ability to practice magic. Priestesses cast their spells according to the phase of the moon and also by their own inner moon phases.

Increase Your Psychic Ability

Mary was clairvoyant. She had dreams about her future and saw angels at least twice in her life, according to the Bible. The first time was when the angel Gabriel came to her and told her she was carrying the baby Jesus. Gabriel is the archangel of communication. She brings messages from the spiritual realm regarding the future and she can help you with your spiritual sight. She will help you to see auras and to see into the future—to see visions, she will also give you clarity and help you to see a situation that has been bugging you from a spiritual perspective.

Today, some traditions teach that Gabriel is a male angel. However, up until the Ecumenical Council during the time of Constantine, Gabriel was regarded as a female angel by Christians. At the Council she was given a sex change and it was decreed she was male. Renaissance paintings depict her as a female and if you work with her, she will probably appear as a woman. Gabriel will open doors for you and help create opportunities in your life to bring your dreams about.

The Fine Art of Seeing Auras

One of the best ways to begin to increase your clairvoyance is to practice seeing auras. An aura is the energy field that vibrates from all things. Everything is made up of energy. Scientists can measure the energy field of any object, animate or inanimate. Our spirit bodies are pure energy and vibrate at different rates, depending on what emotion we are feeling. Each emotion has a different frequency. Low- level emotions like anger, depression, resentment, and envy vibrate at different levels than high-level emotions like joy, love, motivation, and happiness.

Whatever you are vibrating, you will attract to you. This is the law of attraction: like attracts like. By now you know your thoughts are energy, too. So what are you vibrating at this moment and is it something you want to attract more of into your life? Like a magnet, whatever it is you are vibrating, you'll attract more of it to you. This is why it is so important to take responsibility for your thoughts and your feelings so you can begin to consciously attract more of what you *do* want in your life and less of what you don't want.

Most people can see auras through practice and even those who can't see them can usually sense them. Artists have painted auras for centuries. Pictures of saints and the holy trinity are often depicted with their auras shining bright around their heads.

The density and color of an aura depends on the person's health, their mood, their state of mind, and their general disposition. You can learn a lot about a person by observing their aura.

You can learn how to strengthen your own aura, too. Your aura protects you from a variety of outside energies, such as other people's moods or feelings, in much the same way as your skin protects your organs and skeleton. Think of your aura as the protective tissue surrounding your emotional and spiritual body. When your aura is strong and healthy you are less likely to be drained or hurt by other people's thoughts or emotions.

How to See An Aura

First you need to know what you are looking for, so do this exercise at nighttime for the first time. Light a candle in a darkened room and stare at the flame for a few minutes. Notice the almost transparent band of light around the flame; see how it flickers as the flame flickers. If you gently blow the flame the light will move, too, maybe a nanosecond later. If you pick up the candle and move it quickly from one hand to the other, notice how the light around the flame moves. This light looks and moves very much like a human aura. This light is also very much like the energy of angels, fairies, and spirit beings. As you practice seeing auras, you can also practice looking for angels and fairies, too. Sometimes it is easier to see them out of the corner of your eyes or when your eyes are half-closed and your focus is fuzzy. This is because you are using your spiritual sight, not just your physical sight. In fact, if you want to use your spiritual sight alone you can even see them when your physical eyes are closed. They show up like images on a dark screen.

To see a human aura, get a friend to stand against a wall with a plain background. It is easier to see an aura at night because sunlight tends to detract from the light of the aura. Make sure the light in the room is dim. Squint your eyes and stand back from your friend by about three feet, then gaze at the area between her shoulders and around her head. After a while you will begin to see her aura like a faint band of light surrounding her. Get your friend to move side to side and you will notice the aura moves with her—that way you can be assured you don't just have eyeburn!

If you can't see anything, don't worry—keep trying. You can also practice feeling the aura, as some people find this easier to begin with.

Feeling the Aura

Rub your hands together rapidly and then hold them about a foot apart facing each other. Slowly bring them together until you can feel an energy force emitting from them. This will feel like you are holding two magnets toward each other. This is what the aura feels like.

Now rub your hands together and stand close to your friend. Hold your hands above her head or around her shoulders about six inches away. Slowly lower them until you feel a similar magnetlike sensation that you felt before. You can now feel her aura.

Sensing the Aura

Stare hard at the area above your friend's head for a couple of minutes. Try not to think about anything in particular, just look at what you can see. Now close your eyes and notice the first impressions that come to you. You may sense colors, images, or words. Write down these impressions on a piece of paper. Write quickly for three minutes without lifting your hand from the paper to think or edit.

Mary's Glamour

- Soft silver slippers, so you can move soundlessly across the room like the moon moves across the sky

- Magenta, indigo, or purple clothes

- Magenta lip gloss

- Moonstone earrings

- Pearl necklaces

- White clothes with a metallic sheen

Makeup

Line your eyes with sparkly blue eyeliner. Apply a pearly cream eye shadow across your eyelids. Use a pale foundation and apply luminescent highlighter to your forehead and across the top of your cheekbones—you could try "Skinlights" by Revlon. Draw a crescent moon with blue eyeliner on your forehead. Use an opalescent lip gloss or sparkly pale pink lipstick on your lips. Apply lots of ebony mascara to your eyelashes.

Clothing

Dress in a sparkly white dress with a blue cape, shawl, or scarf across your shoulders. Clasp with a silver brooch.

An alternative is to wear a long dress in magenta or purple—these are the colors of the Moon Goddess, too. Or you could try a black or midnight-blue net sheath with silver glitter in it.

For jewelry, try white pearls or moonstone, silver necklaces and rings. For perfume, use honeysuckle or jasmine—flowers whose scents increase during the night. They will increase your psychic receptivity.

Ceremony

Soak in a warm bath for twenty minutes at night. Add a few drops of sandalwood essential oil to the water. Turn the lights off and light a candle and slip into the water. Just relax and imagine all your stress from the day leaking out of you into the water. Let yourself be nurtured by the fragrance. Talk to the Moon Goddess in your mind.

When you get out, put some moisturizer on your skin, dress in your goddess clothing, and apply your makeup. Smudge a little Vicks Vapor Rub in the middle of your forehead to stimulate your third eye and increase your psychic abilities.

Say a prayer to Mary:

Dearest Goddess

Beloved mother Mary

I ask that you

Open my inner vision

So I may see clearly

That which I most need to see

Thank you, dear Goddess

Get a black bowl and fill it three-fourths full with water. Put on some relaxing music and begin to draw in magical energy. Close your eyes and stand with your arms outstretched. Imagine you are pulling in energy from the moon and the stars and from Mary. Feel the magical power filling your body. Ask the archangel Gabriel to be present, too.

Softly chant: "All the magic I need is within me now!" Chant this for three minutes, feeling the power building within you.

Sit on the floor with the bowl of water in front of you. It needs to be a dark color so you can see images in it. Ask Mary a question and see if you can divine the answer in the bowl of water. Squint your eyes like you did in the aura-seeing exercise. Ask Gabriel to give you any information that would best serve you at this time. Close your eyes and see what comes up on your mental movie screen. Write down your experience in your goddess journal. Ask Gabriel to bless your dreams tonight.

You can use this glamour when you want to be more alluring. After invoking Mary, go out and use your moon powers to enchant and mesmerize others.

301

Mary's Tasks for You

* Gaze at the moon for fifteen minutes each night. This is an ancient magical technique to increase your psychic powers. Talk to the Moon Goddess as you do.

* Read the book *Moon Magic* by Dion Fortune (Weiser, 1979). When Dion wrote this book, it was illegal to write nonfiction books about magic, so she put her magical techniques into her novels. This is a wonderful book for learning more about becoming a moon priestess.

* Spend a day as Mary. How does it feel to be a Moon Goddess? Write about it in your goddess journal.

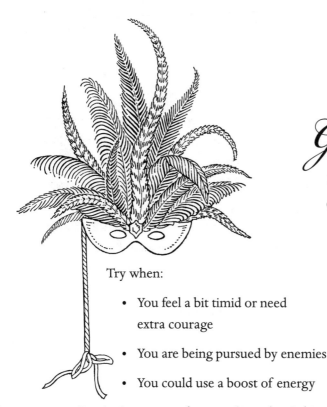

Grania

THE SUN GODDESS

Try when:

- You feel a bit timid or need extra courage

- You are being pursued by enemies

- You could use a boost of energy

Grania (pronounced *gran-yah*) is the Celtic sun goddess. In this chapter we discuss two different Granias who share similar qualities. One is the Celtic sun goddess who was betrothed to an old warrior named Finn. She left him at the altar and ran off with one of his most trusted warriors, the young and gorgeous Diarmid. This story can be seen as a play on the seasonal myths of the sun choosing a young man (representing the spring and summer blaze) over an older man (representing the winter and fall seasons).

The second Grania is Grania O'Malley, an Irishwoman who lived in the sixteenth century. This Grania was a pirate and, like any good Sun Goddess, had a fiery, passionate nature. She fought for her beliefs throughout her life and was a trailblazer during her time.

Grania's Story

The love affair of Grania and Diarmid

Once upon a time, a long, long time ago, there lived a beautiful but headstrong young princess named Grania. Grania lived with her mother and father, the high queen and king of the whole of Ireland, in their castle at Tara.

Grania was the most beautiful of all of King Cormac's daughters, and she was the most lighthearted. As such she had been spoiled shamelessly since she was a child, for whenever she walked into the room it seemed as though she brought the rays of the midsummer sun with her and everyone basked in her sunny glow. It was almost impossible to refuse her any request, such was the strength of her warm, sunny nature.

On this particular day, great excitement filled the halls of Tara, for Finn, the man whose hand had been promised in marriage to Grania, was about to arrive. The castle hustled and bustled with preparations for the great feast. Every nook was cleaned, every pot prepared. For many days the cook had been organizing the kitchen and creating sumptuous dishes for the feast. The aroma of fine meats and honeyed mead filled the castle with its tantalizing smell.

Grania paced nervously in her quarters, awaiting the call from her father to join the party in the great hall. Her mother brushed her fine yellow hair and marveled at the girl before her.

"Oh, Grania, how exciting! This is to be your wedding feast."

"But mother, what if I do not like him?"

"Then you will not be forced into marriage with him, my love," reassured her mother. "Though your father wishes this marriage very much, for Finn is the finest warrior in all of Erin and he commands the Fianna, as you know—the finest warriors in the land. We owe much to Finn for keeping our people safe."

The queen stepped back and gave Grania an appraising look—her body was shapely if not slightly overweight. "Thank goodness women are not fined for being overweight like the men are," she thought, "for Grania is used to a life of luxury and has never had to work a day in her life." Pride filled her heart as she looked upon her daughter's face, for it seemed the sun shone radiantly from the

girl's countenance. Even her head was round like the sun itself, with her long yellow hair falling like sunbeams upon her shoulders. Grania had a heart of gold and
the queen hoped that Finn would warm to this young woman like old bark to a
winter's fire.

Finally the king summoned Grania to the great hall. Her eyes fell immediately
toward Finn, for his stature was immense and his long grey hair sparkled like silver
moonbeams across a black velvet sky. His dark eyes took her in and held her measure. She, too, returned the penetrating stare, unwilling to falter under his gaze. "If
he does not please me," she thought silently, "I shall not marry him. He may be
testing me with his eyes but let me test his presence of mind." For Grania was no
fool in spite of her youth.

Three questions Grania put to Finn, and three questions he answered.

"Who are you, Finn MacCool? I have heard the stories of your bravery in battle, but who is this man before me?"

"I am a warrior," he replied. "And a poet, and a man in need of a wife to fill
my castle with her warmth and love."

"And are you a skilled lover, my lord?" she asked.

Finn was taken back by her bluntness but years of warrior training forced him
to not betray his emotions with his body.

"I know how to please a woman," he stated squarely, looking her in the eyes.

Grania felt a shiver of anticipation run down her spine, for despite the nature
of her questioning, she had yet to lie with a man.

"If you don't give me enough pleasure, I am within my rights by law to take
another lover, you know."

"Yes," agreed Finn. "That you can, but any man you choose has to be of the
same rank as me, so our children will be equal."

"Well, then, Finn MacCool, I will agree to be your wife," said Grania, thinking
it would not be so bad to be rich and live in luxury for the rest of her days. Plus
Finn was the most famous warrior in all of Ireland—something no other man
could boast of.

And with that, the wedding party was seated. Throughout the evening strange
pangs of doubt began to surface through Grania's mind. Finn might be rich, she

thought, and he was certainly a man of high rank and honor. But what had she done, committing herself to this man she barely knew? And as the evening wore on, she saw signs of his age: lines across his forehead, weathered hands that lifted the chalice of mead up to his lips. She imagined those weathered hands stroking her body and, to be honest, the thought repulsed her.

Raucous laughter broke her thoughts and she looked toward the table from where it came. Seated across the hall was a group of young men. There were several young warriors from the Fianna, laughing and joking and merrymaking. Grania wished she could go and join them. One in particular caught her attention. A young man of about twenty, his brown hair streaked with gold, who was tall and lean and his eyes lit up as if illuminated with sunlight, shining brightly on those around him. All the others at the table seemed to be paying particular attention to him, and, Grania noticed, the girls at the nearby tables seemed to hang on his every word.

"Mother?" she queried, tugging her mother's sleeve. "Who is that young man with the shining eyes and the delightful smile?"

"Oh, Grania," sighed her mother. "Why, that is Diarmid. He is a fine young warrior, one of the bravest in all of the Fianna. But don't you look at him like that, for you are already spoken for—you gave your word. Diarmid is a fine young man but remember, he is honor bound to Finn, and anyway he has plenty of women willing to throw themselves at him. Diarmid never lacks for company in his bed. Surely you do not wish to be another notch in his belt?"

However, Grania had heard of the legendary lover Diarmid. His reputation surpassed him and she knew he was honor bound to never refuse the request of a woman due to a magical command placed on him years earlier.

"Let's see how brave you really are," she thought to herself, a plan already taking shape in her mind.

Grania eased herself over to where Diarmid was standing.

"Diarmid?" she asked. "Is it true that you must never refuse the request of a woman?"

Diarmid looked at this woman before him—it was not the first time that night he had noticed Grania, for every man in the hall had glanced surreptitiously at her throughout the evening, envying Finn the chance to make her his bride. Her beauty surpassed her, for it was not so much her physical attributes that made her attractive but the warm glow of sunlight that surrounded her as she moved through the crowd.

Diarmid replied carefully, "I am honor bound to never refuse the request of a woman in need, that is true. But an honorable woman would never make a request unless it was truly serious."

"Then take me away from here. Far, far away—for I do not wish to marry Finn. He is too old!" she said emphatically.

Diarmid stared at her, shocked. "I cannot take you away, Grania, for my loyalty lies with Finn. I cannot break my oath as a warrior. I am sorry."

"Oh, yes, you can!" replied Grania. "I am a woman, and I am in need! I do not want to marry an old man. You must take me away from here!"

"Not as long as my life is worth living!" said Diarmid.

"You must, you are honor bound!"

"Grania, you are very beautiful and I am truly flattered that you would want me to take you, but I can't," whispered Diarmid gently.

"You must," insisted Grania, "for you are honor bound."

Diarmid sighed. He knew he was caught. "Very well, then, we shall go. But Finn will be furious when he learns of our departure. We must run far, far away."

The two slipped out into the warm summer evening. When Finn discovered their departure some hours later, he was indeed furious. He ordered all the men under his command to search for the two. His fury held no bounds. How dare Grania disgrace him in front of all his men, and how dare one of his own warriors betray him as such!

For many months Grania and Diarmid ran and hid from Finn and his men. It was not safe for them to hide at other castles among people so they became fugitives, sleeping outdoors in hollows and under trees wherever they could. As they went, they foraged for food—nuts and berries from the bushes, salmon from the rivers, and whatever other gifts the Earth Mother would bestow on them.

Grania longed to sleep with Diarmid, for his beauty was mesmerizing; however, he refused her time and time again. "I have done what you asked of me,

307

Grania, ask no more," he said. "For I will not betray Finn in that way, too." And each morning after they awoke, Diarmid placed a piece of unbroken bread in their wake as a sign to Finn that he had not slept with Grania.

Diarmid's honor only served to make him more desirable to Grania, who had fallen in love with the handsome young man who was her protector and now her only friend.

As the months turned into years, Grania grew tired and weary of being always on the run. Her impetuous decision no longer seemed quite so adventurous. She was tired and lonely for her friends and longed to go home. But going home was no longer an option. She knew Diarmid would be killed for his actions and she could not live with herself if that were to happen. Even if she explained it was all her idea, Finn would have to kill him to save face.

The firelight glowed in their campsite. Grania looked at Diarmid. How tired he looked. "This is not easy on him, either," she thought. For now she no longer thought only of herself but of the consequences of her actions on others.

Diarmid had given up everything for her—his honor, his friends, his family, his clan, and his warrior brotherhood, which had been a source of great pride to him. Sadness filled her heart. How selfish she had been. He had not even wanted to go with her. He had not even eloped with her from love. And what had she to show for it? An aching heart, a strong, sinewy body, and the knowledge her life would never be the same again.

Diarmid glanced up and caught Grania's eye. He saw the pain in them and his heart went out to her, for Grania was not the spoiled young girl who had first demanded he must run away with her. He marveled at the way she had adjusted to living on the run—she who had been used to every luxury was now adept at fending for herself. Her body was strong and sculpted from months of hard work—but so, too, was her character. She was no longer the impetuous child he had first met.

And Diarmid thought her more beautiful than he did when he had first laid eyes on her. Her spirit glowed like a dozen rainbows lit up by thirteen suns.

She walked toward him tentatively at first, as if unsure whether he would once again turn her away. Her steps became more confident the closer she got. He held her gaze. No words were spoken; none were needed as he took her hand and made love to her from the bottom of his heart.

The next morning he left a piece of broken bread for all to see.

Goddess Workout

Grania's story is very close to my own heart, for I was Grania in a play that my friend Maya Sutton produced. Maya's retelling of the story gave me a greater glimpse into the character of Grania and how she matured over the years. For seven years (some myths say sixteen), she and Diarmid were on the run until finally Finn caught them.

Grania starts out wanting something so badly that she doesn't think of the long-term consequences. She has no thoughts of those around her and how her actions will affect them, too. Have you ever felt like that? Like the sun, Grania was warm and fun to be around, but too much sun without protection can lead to getting burned.

Here are some questions for you to ponder.

Do you think Grania was wrong or right in her decision to elope with Diarmid? Why?

What might you have done in similar circumstances?

What could have been a better way for Grania to get what she wanted without causing those around her to suffer?

When have you ever acted impetuously without thinking through your actions? What were the consequences?

309

The Ten Degrees of Celtic Marriage

In Celtic society, marriage was polyamorous and men and women could take several lovers. The Brehon laws were the main legal system that was used when the Celts were at the height of their power, from about 500 B.C. to A.D. 500.

Any relationship that resulted in the birth of a child was considered to be a marriage in Celtic society under the Brehon laws. In this way women's rights were protected and no child was illegitimate. By law both parents were responsible for raising a child. However, if the child was the result of rape or of adultery, then the man was solely responsible for raising the child. The woman also received monetary compensation for the rape. Celtic laws were based on compensation rather than capital punishment. If the woman was unsure who had raped her, she received compensation from the king. Also, if the woman was sick, then the sole responsibility of the child's welfare fell onto the father.

The Celts had ten different types of marriage, not just one like in our society today.

First-degree marriage took place between partners of equal status and property. Grania's marriage to Finn would have been a first-degree marriage.

Second-degree marriage was when the man had more property and supported the woman.

Third-degree marriage was when the woman had more property and wealth than the man—with the added stipulation that the man must agree to till his wife's fields or manage her cattle in order to keep her dignity and respect.

Fourth-degree marriage was different—it was in effect a love marriage, and the woman was in effect a concubine. The rights of the children were described and safeguarded by law, but if the husband died the woman had to return to her kin.

Marriage of the fifth degree was when two people had sex but lived in separate dwellings.

Sixth-degree marriage was when a woman was taken against her will or abducted, like when a warrior would take the wife of his enemy after he had defeated him in battle. He was married to her for as long as he could keep her with him!

Seventh-degree marriage was a one-night stand, also known as "a soldier's marriage" because warriors would often have this kind of union! If a child resulted, then he or she would have the status and rank of the father. A warrior was considered of high class in Celtic society.

Eighth-degree marriage was when a man seduced a woman through deception, such as telling her lies about his status or his property, or getting her drunk so he could sleep with her, taking advantage of her intoxication.

An act of rape constituted the ninth-degree marriage.

And the tenth-degree marriage was a marriage that took place between two feeble-minded people or intellectually challenged people.

311

Women's Rights In Celtic Society
(circa 500 B.C.–A.D. 500)

Just as Grania stated in her story, a married woman could legally take a lover if she was dissatisfied with her husband's sexual performance. Plus, men were fined for being overweight in Celtic society. This was because they were a warrior race and the welfare and wealth of the tribes depended on the prowess of their warriors.

Women in Celtic society enjoyed more sexual freedom and freedom in general than women in our society probably do today! They certainly had more freedom than their Greek or Roman contemporaries.

Roman women could only leave the house if they were accompanied by their spouse or a brother or father, and they could go shopping and visit theaters and law courts only if they wore a special outfit. Roman women could also take part in their husband's business discussions with associates at dinnertime. Roman men ruled their households and had ultimate authority over their women—wives and daughters.

Greek women were not allowed to even be present at the dinner table with the men unless it was a family dinner party. Most of the time they were relegated to a remote part of the house, called a gynaeceum. Women could not own property and were considered the property of first their fathers and then their husbands.

By law a Celtic woman could own property, which they would not be deprived of even when they got married. They could hold high positions in politics, religions, and the arts—they could govern and rule, have careers in politics, be war leaders, judges, priests, and lawmakers. They could get divorced if they chose and if they were deserted, molested, or mistreated, they could claim considerable financial remuneration.

Here are some of the things Celtic women were entitled to by law:

- Equal pay for equal work

- Wages for housework (I wish this was still the case!)

- Protection from violence

- Fair separation laws so that they got a fair amount of wealth and property

- Both spouses were required by law to respect one another; they could be fined if they acted derisively toward one another

A woman could divorce her husband for any number of reasons, including smelly breath! Men were fined if they physically assaulted a woman and if they verbally assaulted her, too!

Here are some examples of verbal assaults, which were illegal and subject to monetary compensation for the woman:

- Mocking a woman's appearance

- Making derisory comments about a physical defect

- Taunting, teasing, and name-calling

- Repeating stories about her that weren't true

Celtic women were free to choose their husbands and lovers openly. If her husband was infertile, she could go away to "seek a child." If she became pregnant by another man, the baby was treated as the child of her husband.

Even as the Celtic lands became Christianized, Celtic women could still preach and give Mass. However, as time went on, the laws were changed so women were gradually stripped of their independence. It was the Christians who brought punishments such as the death penalty, mutilation, and flogging to Celtic society.

Grania Ni Mhaille, the Irish Pirate Queen

Grania Ni Mhaille or Grania O'Malley was an Irish pirate who lived in the sixteenth century—and she rocked! Just like Grania in the myth, Grania the pirate was headstrong and independent. She had an infamous career as a pirate and commanded three pirate ships with two hundred men under her, and fought against the English who were trying to subjugate Ireland at the time. Grania was from the county of Connaught and she had many storms to face, both political and personal, as well as the ones on the high seas.

Grania sailed her pirate ships from Clew Bay in Ireland to Scotland and England and even as far away as Spain and Portugal. She was married twice: the first time when she was sixteen to Donal O'Flaherty, who was a well-known warrior. Donal was murdered by the Joyces, a neighboring clan, who then tried to take possession of his castle. But Grania rallied her husband's clan together and fought back until the Joyces retreated. She had three children while married to Donal and by the time she was in her thirties she was a widow without any financial rights. So Grania got men from neighboring clans to join her army and set sail as pirates. This was an amazing feat as at that time Ireland was not a unified country like England but consisted of as many as sixty counties, each with their own clans and ruling chieftains. There was no central leader of Ireland like England, which had Queen Elizabeth I. The clans in Ireland were often feuding with one another so for men to leave their own clan and follow Grania says a lot about her personality.

A pirate's life was physically demanding as well as dangerous. Grania needed many skills to develop her career. She had a great knowledge of ships and sailing. She could fire a musket and fight for her crew. She could navigate through treacherous waters and use the stars as a guide as well as a compass. She knew the lands and routes like the back of her hand. She had to be able to foretell the weather and gauge the mood of the sea. She was responsible for the lives and livelihood of two hundred men as well as her own family. Her fourth child, Tibbot, was born at sea and the next day Grania fought with her men against Algerian pirates!

Piracy was illegal and you would be hung if convicted. Living conditions on the ships were harsh. Violence, gambling, poor hygiene, swearing, partying, and lack of privacy and space were a way of life—not to mention calloused skin. Grania had a successful pirate career for forty years. However, she had many enemies, not only other pirates out at sea but also the English, who were trying to curtail her power, and other Irish clans who fought against her, too.

By the time she was sixty-three in 1593 she had been through a lot. Here are some of the things Grania endured:

- Her first husband was murdered by the Joyces.

- Her eldest son was killed.

- Her ships, cattle, and horses were confiscated by the English.

- Her lands in Connaught were devastated by war.

- She had been in jail for two years.

- Her wealth and rights were stripped from her.

- A boyfriend, whom she was deeply in love with, was killed.

- Her movements were restricted and she was hounded by her enemies.

- One of her sons pledged his loyalty to the English.

The fact that she was even alive at sixty-three was amazing, as the average life span at that time was fifty for a woman. So here she was sixty-three, broke, a widow for the second time and without a way to make money because the English had curtailed her activities. But did Grania sit back and give up? No way. She went to England to talk to Queen Elizabeth.

Grania bowed to nobody. She was a leader. She was courageous, persistent, and determined.

Grania was not a woman to mess with. Once she tried to starve to death another chieftain who had crossed her by trying to steal her property. And another time she kidnapped the grandson of a lord who was rude to her when she visited his castle. For ransom she demanded he be more hospitable to his guests and always keep an extra place set at his table in case of company.

Irish Women in the Sixteenth Century

By the time Grania Ni Mhaille was born about A.D. 1530 the Celtic laws had changed dramatically. When Celtic society was at its most powerful there were many warrior women, both in legend and in history—women like Queen Maeve, who was also from Connaught, and Scathach from the Isle of Skye, and Queen Boadicea from the Iceni tribe. However, when Grania was born it was very unusual to be a career woman, much less a warrior, a ruler, a military commander, and a political activist, although the day-to-day activities were still much the same—clans still fought against each other and cattle was the primary currency.

The influx of the English to Ireland and their Christian Roman laws had changed women's lives dramatically.

Ireland was the only Celtic land the Romans never conquered before the demise of the Roman Empire. But when Saint Patrick came to Ireland in the fifth century A.D. he introduced Christianity and the Roman Salic laws. When Rome accepted Christianity as its main religion, each country it conquered was then required to accept it, too. Roman Salic law was very different from the old Celtic Brehon laws. Over time the Brehon laws became replaced with more and more of the Roman laws, and Celtic women were gradually stripped of their previous rights.

By the sixteenth century, Irish women were pretty much relegated to having babies and taking care of the households. Even the wives of chieftains, who were the upper class, could no longer run for government or be lawyers. Their main claim to fame was to do charity work, housework, keep the maintenance of the castle in order, organize feasts for their husband's allies, and raise the children. Occasionally they would do a bit of informal teaching, too.

However, there were some rights that women still retained, like the right to keep their maiden name once they married, and the right to own property and land, and they could still divorce their husbands. Also handfasting marriages still existed from earlier times. Couples could have a trial marriage for a year and a day and then decide if they wanted to stay together for longer. When Grania married her second husband, Richard Burke, she made sure she had a prenuptial agreement that said she could keep her property and wealth if they divorced.

Navigating Through the Storms In Your Life

I wish I could tell you your life was going to be fabulous every day from this point forward, but that is probably not the case. As my friend Harvey says, life can't be lollipops all the time. Sometimes you go through the school of hard knocks and emerge stronger on the other side. Chances are some of you will probably get your heart broken several times, get rejected in work and in love as you go through life, fail miserably at something important, and have to deal with some pretty tough situations.

Like Grania, you may have many storms to face, but I want you to know it is not so much the difficulty of the storms but learning how to navigate through them that is the important thing. You've got to know that you are bigger than any problem or situation you might face, and that you have the tenacity and courage to cope. You've got to learn that you can heal a broken heart, deal with a great tragedy, and cope with whatever life hands you—good or bad. Unfortunately the way to such knowledge is often from overcoming hardships. But rest assured the reward for your pain is strength of character and absolute trust in your ability to care for yourself.

I used to wish bad stuff wouldn't happen—I wanted a nice cruisy life. But I have had my fair share of knocks, just like everybody, and I wouldn't trade a minute of them. I grew up with a bipolar mother, never knowing at nighttime if she was going to burst through my bedroom door and get violent with me. I had to deal with my mother's death by drug overdose, getting raped at a party, lots of abusive boyfriends, business rejections, and, like everyone else, lots of other stuff.

But as my husband says, we all have miles and miles of crap behind us. I know that I wouldn't be the woman I am today if it weren't for those events. Those experiences shaped my character and made me who I am. And you know what? I kind of like who I am. I'm not perfect by any stretch of the imagination, but I'm okay. And for whatever difficult situation you encounter, I want you to know that you will be okay, too. I have great faith in you. We are not wimpy women—we are Goddess Women and, like Grania, we can draw on great reservoirs of divine courage and persistence in the face of adversity.

I think our society has a tendency to teach us sometimes that we are fragile, and this does us a great disservice. We must stop thinking of ourselves as wounded and permanently emotionally disfigured when tragedy hits. Instead we must create a blueprint of ourselves as strong, healthy warrior women—women who live full lives that consist of great tragedy and great joy. In Celtic society, scars were considered beauty marks—so wear your beauty marks with pride.

Signposts Through the Storm

Find a role model who has been through what you are going through and has not only survived but is thriving. Even if this is not someone you personally know but someone that you read about, it is very helpful to know that someone else has been through the same stuff and can reassure you that you will be okay and give you gentle guidance.

Face Your Pain Head-On

There may be situations where you feel a great deal of loss, grief, hurt, and pain. Don't try to numb it out with drugs or alcohol, or by running away from it. Both the Granias encountered a lot of pain. Grania O'Malley's husband was executed— she had to deal with the pain of losing him by something totally unjust and unfair. Her lover was also murdered. Don't be afraid of emotional pain. As a human you have a capacity to feel great pain and to feel great joy. Pain itself will not kill you. It may feel like it will sometimes, but it won't. What you do with the pain can be destructive or constructive. If you need help, find a professional or a friend or mentor who can help steer you in the right direction.

Create Your Own Definition of What Is Possible— Don't Listen to the Odds or the "Experts"

Sometimes statistics can make you feel worse rather than better. There seem to be statistics and experts for everything, from how long it takes to heal from a tragedy to how likely it is that your boyfriend will cheat on you and what the odds are of your being successful in your chosen career.

You've got to decide when you hear statistics or statements whether they are things that you want to be true for you or not. Do you want them to be part of your belief system, or do you want to believe in something larger? Even if someone has never done something before, it doesn't mean it can't be done.

Know That You Absolutely Have the Ability to Heal from Anything

Our bodies, minds, and spirits are amazing in their ability to heal. Healing doesn't always mean curing. There's a difference. Last year two of my friends had cancer. One died and one lived—but they both healed, even though they had very different outcomes.

You can heal any situation in your life with the divine power of the Goddess.

Think of Yourself as a Pioneer Woman

Grania was a pioneer woman in her time. She forged what was previously considered impossible for a woman to do in her lifetime. This country was built on the courage of pioneer women. Pioneer blood runs in your veins no matter what country you hail from. All pioneer women encounter adversity. You will, too—see it as a challenge to push you further forward rather than a sign that you may as well give up.

Create a Vision of Your Future Self as Healthy and Whole

Close your eyes and see a picture of your future self in your imagination. Make it as many years in the future as feels right to you—one year, two years, five, or ten. See her as happy, empowered, and living the kind of life you dream about. See her as putting the past completely behind her, having gained the lessons learned and having left all the bad stuff behind. See her radiant and smiling. Keep building this picture up in your imagination.

Receive Energy from Your Future Self—
See a Link from Her to You

Now see your future self sending energy back to you to help you heal today. See her stretching out her arms in love to you and sending light from her heart center to your heart center. Whenever you feel like you can't make it through the day, call out to your future self, close your eyes, and connect to her with a beam of light.

Tune Into Your Goddess Self—Make Your Aura Much Bigger
than Any Problem You Might Encounter

Your divine self is much larger than any situation you will ever encounter. When lightning strikes and you feel your world spinning out of control, create a vision of yourself in your mind's eye as being much larger than any event that can possibly happen to you. See your aura as forty feet high and forty feet wide, and see the event as tiny in comparison. See yourself as much larger and more magnificent than the event.

Sometimes when storms hit we tend to feel tiny against them, like a little ship in a great big tumultuous ocean. Turn it around in your imagination and see your goddess self as this great big luminescent being with a brilliant sparkling aura that radiates outward from your heart center.

Bring Light to the Situation—
Sunlight, Starlight, Moonlight, Divine Light

Imagine a hole in the top of your head. Now close your eyes and imagine divine light being funneled through this hole into every cell in your being. Flood your body, your mind, and your emotions with divine light. Imagine light from the stars, the sun, and the moon being transmitted to you right now. Imagine the situation, the other people involved, and the place where it happened being flooded with light, too.

Ask Grania to Pour Her Sunlight On It

See Grania pouring divine sunlight onto the situation. Ask her to fill you with her divine power and courage. Ask her what she would do in a similar situation. Spend some time hanging out with Grania in your imagination—Grania the pirate or Grania the sun goddess, or both of them!

Watch the Pictures In Your Head

Our minds have a tendency to want to replay situations over and over again. If you have been through a traumatic event, like rape, for example, and you keep playing it over and over in your head three times a day for a year, then that is over a thousand times that you relive the trauma. Remember, your subconscious mind can't tell the difference between something you vividly imagine and something that is actually happening. So create a pattern interruption whenever you start replaying the event in your mind. You can absolutely train your mind to think about other things.

Imagine the Situation as You Would Like It to Have Been

Using rape as our example again, imagine the situation as you wish it had been. Maybe you wish it had never happened, so create what you would have liked to happen instead in your imagination. Or create a vision of yourself beating the crap out of the person who attacked you. If you got rejected in love, imagine yourself finding someone better who loves you deeply—use your imagination in wise and creative ways. You will create new neuroassociations or pathways in your brain to help you move forward. Remember, each time you think about something vividly in your mind that's the way your body will experience it, too. So create fun fantasies to focus on.

Send Healing Energy Into the Past

Close your eyes and imagine divine light radiating from your heart back into the past. See the whole situation enshrined in light. Know that you absolutely have the power to bring light to all the dark places in your heart, your body, and your life—past, present, or future.

320

Blend with the Power of the Goddess

Know you can do anything with the power of the Goddess. Divine power is strong, powerful, wise, loving, and kind.

Have Some Fun!

Take some time out to do something fun, just for you. Do one thing each day that makes you happy.

The Similarities Between the Two Granias

Here are some similarities between the two Granias, even though one was from myth and one was a real person.

- They were both stubborn. Neither of them accepted the rules of how they should behave according to their society.

- They were both persistent. They each had a vision of what they wanted to accomplish and they didn't give up when the going got tough.

- They were both courageous. Each woman was pursued by her enemies and had to develop strong strategies for not being caught. They fought for what they wanted and what they believed in.

- They both suffered devastating losses. Grania from myth lost her family, her friends, and all her familiar surroundings, and eventually she lost Diarmid at the hands of Finn, too. Grania O'Malley lost two husbands, a lover, her freedom, and eventually her battle against the English. Does this mean that they would have been better off not even fighting for what they wanted? No, because what they achieved during their lifetimes was far greater than the sum of their losses.

- They both came up against attack and learned how to navigate in the wilderness of their lives.

Grania's Glamour

- "Pirate" outfit—jeans, shirt, and vest

- Golden hoop earrings

- Cargo pants with floral T-shirts

- Gold sparkly lip gloss

Makeup

Line your eyes with forest green eyeliner and dust copper eye shadow over your eyelids. Wear a tinted moisturizer with SPF 15 to protect your skin from the sun. Keep your makeup fresh and natural looking. Both these goddesses were practical women who led physically demanding lives. They were aware of their feminine power and what they could accomplish.

Clothing

Try cargo pants or jeans, or striped pants with a floral T-shirt and denim jacket. Wear clothes that are comfortable and that you can move easily in.

Ceremony

Close your eyes and imagine both Granias are standing before you. From their hearts they are radiating energy to your heart. You see the energy as a beam of light like a sunbeam—the beam is strong, steady, and consistent. Grania the pirate queen tells you they will send you three divine qualities—courage, determination, and persistence. She asks you to get comfortable, to breathe deeply, and be receptive to the divine energy they are sending you.

First they send you a laser beam of courage. You feel this divine courage entering your body through your heart. It fills your entire body and radiates outward.

Next they send you a light beam of determination. Again you feel the divine power of determination filling your veins. In your mind's eye you see yourself finishing an important task.

Last they send you a beam of persistence. You feel the divine power of persistence radiating through your heart and throughout your body. Notice if the three qualities they have sent you feel different as you embody them. Say the words *courage, determination,* and *persistence* over and over in your mind until you feel your energy grow strong and determined.

Grania the pirate looks into your eyes and says, "You need never fear your enemies. No one can hurt you without your consent. People might physically injure you but they cannot hurt your feelings unless you already feel doubt in that area. You have the power to deflect other people's hatred and venom. You don't have to accept it if that is what they are sending you. You can block it with your mind and breathe it out of your aura.

"Know that you have the power to keep other people's energy separate from your own. Feel your own energy as a warm vibrating sun within your heart center. See this sun shining brightly and sending out sunlight in all directions. Feel it pulsating brilliantly in your body now."

You see a bright sun in the middle of your chest and focus on how much power it is generating. You know that by tuning into this inner sun you can radiate sunlight to everyone around you and you can increase your own vibrancy and personal power. Whenever you are in the presence of "enemies" you can close your eyes and tune into your own energy center and refuse to take their energy on. The more aware you are of your own energy and vitality, the less likely you will be affected by others. Whenever you are around people who are very strong-minded or domineering, imagine your energy is six times stronger.

Turn up the dial of your inner sun to radiate more light and warmth. With your imagination, practice playing with your inner sunlight, turning the energy up and then bringing it down again. Know that you can choose at any given moment how much energy you want to feel.

Grania's Tasks for You

- Go out into the world as Grania the sun goddess one day this week. Practice radiating sunlight from your heart. How does it feel to be the Sun Goddess? Write about your experiences in your goddess journal.

323

- Think of a situation where you have been procrastinating. Have you been avoiding the tasks out of fear or self-doubt? In your imagination, see yourself bringing divine courage, determination, and persistence to the tasks. See yourself completing them easily and effortlessly, being gently guided by Grania.

- Are there any "enemies" in your life who are hounding you at this time? If so, practice staying in your own energy when you are around them. Don't let them throw you off your center by their bad moods. Practice radiating your own energy at different times during the day.

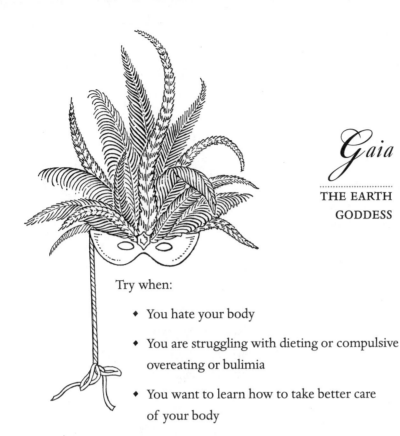

Gaia

....

**THE EARTH
GODDESS**

Try when:

• You hate your body

• You are struggling with dieting or compulsive
overeating or bulimia

• You want to learn how to take better care
of your body

Gaia (pronounced *gay-ah*) is the Greek goddess of the Earth.
Not just a guardian of the Earth, she is the Earth herself, from
whom all life comes and to whom all life returns. In Greek
mythology, Gaia is the mother of all deities as well as the
mother of all life on Earth. Her body is our beloved planet.
The hills and mountains are her breasts, the fields and mead-
ows her body, the rivers and waterfalls her blood. She births
us and sustains us with the plentiful food from her glorious
body. Indeed, she is our beloved mother—lie upon her and listen to her heartbeat, let her soothe and comfort you, seek
refuge and sustenance upon her sacred body.

All that dies, our bodies included, return to her and become nourishment for her fertile soil so the cycle of life can
begin again.

Gaia is the goddess of abundance, earthy sensuality, and fertility. She will show you how to care for your body. She will help you birth your dreams and desires and give them substance and form on Earth, bringing them forth from the invisible spiritual plane into the visible physical world of matter.

If you have any struggles concerning food, love, addictions, compulsive overeating, or constant dieting, Gaia is the goddess who will help you. She will help you heal your relationship with your own body. She weeps every time you look into the mirror and hate what you see, for it is her image you denigrate. She cries out in pain at the millions of women weeping with the shame of their bodies—millions of women struggling to make their bodies barren like a desert, barely just skin and bones. Gaia will set you free.

She will teach you to love your body and value its messages and gifts. She will teach you how to care for your body on a spiritual level, emotional level, and physical level. She will show you how to open up to your own sensuality, for it is through our physical senses we experience much. Gaia nourishes all that lives and that includes you!

Gaia's Story

Gaia, the goddess who births the world

Once upon a time, a long, long time ago, there was a beautiful, large, voluptuous goddess named Gaia. Her body was round and welcoming like the Earth itself. Her hair flowed down her back like a waterfall cascading around her, and her face was so warm and friendly that when she smiled it was as if the sun shone from her, enveloping all in her radiance. Everywhere Gaia walked things flourished, for she was the earth goddess, goddess of birth and growth and prosperity.

Now Gaia lived at the top of Mount Olympus, which was the highest mountain in Greece. She came out of the great Chaos and gave birth to Uranus, the sky god who then became her husband. Their relationship was very passionate. Uranus clasped Gaia to him so tightly, refusing to let go, that the babies in her belly could not emerge from her womb!

However, the youngest one of these children, Cronus, decided to overthrow Uranus so he could free his siblings and himself. Gaia conceived a great sickle within her womb and from in there Cronus cut off his father's penis while it was still inside Gaia. Uranus bellowed so loudly it shook the world, and he lifted his arms in horror. No longer entwined with Gaia, the Earth, he floated upward, settling into his new position so the sky was separate from the Earth.

From Uranus's blood, Gaia also conceived the Furies, the avenging goddesses who pursued murderers. Cronus was the new ruler of the universe and he took his sister Rhea as his bride. There were twelve children conceived by Gaia and Uranus who were freed from Gaia's womb. They were known as the Titans, and they were the first gods and goddesses in Greek mythology. They lived in Olympus, loving and quarreling among themselves and sometimes with mortals. According to their moods, they would help or hinder humans, these golden godly ones.

Now Cronus was as tyrannical as Uranus had been. One of the priestesses at the Oracle of Delphi warned him that he would be replaced by one of his own sons. So each time his wife Rhea bore a child, he would quickly swallow it as soon as it was born.

Rhea longed for a child she could hold in her arms and raise to adulthood, so she sought Gaia's advice.

"Wrap a large stone in a baby's blanket," Gaia suggested. "Then let Cronus swallow that instead of the babe."

So the next time Rhea gave birth, she made sure she had a large stone next to her bed. Before her husband entered, she bade her maid quickly whisk the babe away and she put the stone in the swaddling instead. Cronus entered the room, grabbed the baby bundle, and swallowed the stone without so much as blinking his eyes. And the little baby Zeus was carried away in great secrecy to Crete, where he was raised in safety.

When Zeus was grown up, he returned to Olympus and demanded his father throw up the children he had swallowed. Zeus and Cronus engaged in a bitter battle, with Cronus finally succumbing to Zeus. So Cronus vomited up all the children he had swallowed who were now grown gods and goddesses. These included Zeus's future wife, Hera; Poseidon, the sea god; Demeter, the goddess of vegetation; and Hades, god of the underworld.

And Zeus became the ruler of Olympus in his father's stead. Presently his grandmother Gaia came to him and said, "Zeus, you must beware the same fate does not befall you as befell your father and your grandfather. For you will bear a child by the goddess Metis, and if you are not careful he will overthrow you and replace you as the supreme god."

So Zeus swallowed Metis, whose name means "thought," and later Athena, goddess of wisdom and judgment, sprang from his head.

The story of separation between Earth and sky is an ancient one. It is found in many different cultures, especially in West Asian mythology. While the Greek version may appear quite violent, it is not as violent as the one from the Hurrians, who lived on the border of what is now Turkey and Iraq. In their story, Kumarbi, the equivalent of Cronus, bit off and swallowed his father's penis. However, as a result of his actions, Kumarbi became pregnant with terrifying deities, one of whom overthrew him eventually.

The Earth Goddess

The Earth Goddess will provide you with a strong foundation and a great deal of stability. She will give you patience so you can gestate your dreams, visions, and plans within her fertile soil until they are ready to be born into the world. Physically she will help you replenish and rebuild your body so you can face each day with renewed vigor. Emotionally she will give you stability and a strong sense of self.

Earth People

Like the Earth herself, people with a lot of earth in them are slow to change. They like to stick to one project for a long time and they like a lot of stability in their lives. Change and upheaval feel uncomfortable. They make decisions carefully, putting a lot of time and thought into it before they act. Once they have decided a course of action, they will follow through without being swayed by passing fancies.

Earth people are extremely nurturing and compassionate. They love deeply and don't often get infatuations—they are not fickle with their feelings. Their love is deep and unwavering, with roots planted way beneath what is visible. Earth people are very physical and like to show their affection with lots of hugs and kisses. They like to live in comfortable surroundings, too. They are practical and efficient and make great organizers.

People with a lot of earth in their physical bodies tend to be sturdy and have stocky frames. They are usually medium to large build and have a tendency to gain weight and find it difficult to lose it.

Keeping Earth In Balance

When you have just the right amount of earth, you will be compassionate without being overbearing. You will trust the process of life. You will take care of your physical body and your physical surroundings without being obsessive about it. You will feel self-reliant and know that there is an endless source available to you at all times, that the universe will always provide for you whatever it is that you need.

Too Little Earth

When people don't have enough earth energy, they become restless and flighty, quickly jumping from one thing to another without ever finishing projects. They can be ungrounded and spacey, not very in touch with the physical world.

They seem to live on another planet at times. They can feel alienated, like they don't quite fit in on earth. Not enough earth can lead to forgetfulness and clumsiness. Simple tasks like balancing their checkbooks or buying all the groceries they set out to get can be difficult.

Too Much Earth

People with too much earth can be very materialistic. They cling to possessions and people. They hoard their belongings. They can be bossy and try to control others, thinking they know what is best for everyone. Set in their ways, they can find changing a habit or belief extremely difficult. People with lots of earth are the most stubborn around! Once they have an opinion, they will stick to it, defying any sense of rationality. They are loyal to a fault.

How to Get More Earth

If you have been feeling a little spacey lately or acting too impulsively, you need more earth in your body. Try:

+ Lying outside on the ground for twenty minutes

+ Eating root vegetables that are grown within the earth, like potatoes, carrots, or yams

+ Eating more carbohydrates, like bread, pasta, and rice

+ Finishing a project you have been avoiding doing—ask Gaia to help you follow through

What If You Have Too Much Earth?

If you have too much earth, do things that will loosen you up. Try:

+ Yoga or stretching for ten minutes every day to increase your mental flexibility as well as your physical flexibility

+ Eating foods with a high water content, like lettuce, or eating light foods and going easy on carbohydrates for a few days

+ Doing something spontaneous: change your routine, walk a different way to school, buy a food you have never tried before

Earth Magic

Earth magic involves making the invisible visible, bringing ideas, visions, dreams, and desires into a concrete reality through your actions. (Actions are the realm of the Fire Goddess.) When you look at the four goddesses of the elements they follow a perfect circle: The Air Goddess inspires, the Fire Goddess nudges you to take action, the Water Goddess helps you reflect and refine your actions and channel your passion into your dreams, and the Earth Goddess gifts you with the completed project.

In Her Image

Healing body image with the help of the Goddess and her angels

Body image is the picture you have of your body—what it looks like to you and how you think others see it. Your body image may be accurate or inaccurate, or it may be detailed or vague. It really doesn't matter how "real" your body image is. What matters most is how you feel about your body.

Your image of your body may change according to your mood, your age, the time of the month it is, what the scales say, or if you are bloated, sick, or pregnant. If you are under a lot of stress or have just begun or ended a relationship, your feelings can be reflected in your body image.

A lot of our feelings about our bodies come from the homes in which we are raised and the society in which we live. If you live in a household where you are teased about your size or where your mother has a negative body image, you are likely to develop one, too. Likewise, American media is especially guilty of reinforcing the idea that slim is better, slim is sexier. These ideas oppress women with their unrealistic weight and size expectations. Rarely is there a glimpse of a large-sized happy, healthy, successful woman on TV, in film, or in a fashion magazine—although this trend does seem to be changing. Women become disempowered and restricted by this enslaving attitude force-fed to us by the media. In other Western countries there is more exposure to different sized women. In November 2001, Australian *Cosmopolitan* had a fabulous fashion layout of a very large, very beautiful model surrounded by gorgeous guys. Aussie *Cosmo* often uses large-sized models as well as thin ones. On British TV you see a wide variety of women in leading roles—check out BBC America sometime and see the difference. Attitudes are slowly changing and little by little we are starting to see more magazines and TV shows showing women of all sizes.

What is so damaging about the media's pressure for girls to conform to a certain look is that even the images you see in teen magazines are not real. For every photo you see of a girl model in any major magazine, air brushing and computer touch-ups have removed her pimples, her cellulite, excess skin or flab, and any other "imperfection" that the editor does not want you to see. It is common for eye color to be changed, breasts to be enhanced, or thighs to be downsized—all with one little click of a button on the computer. So what you are seeing when you look at the "perfect girl" in a magazine is not really real anyway! If you are trying to live up to the images you see in magazines, you are trying to live up to something that doesn't really exist. So stop torturing yourself.

The Goddess can help you heal a bad body image. Even if you have spent years hating the way you feel about your body, you can change. Your body is an amazing guide. Through your body you can receive many divine signals. Your body tells you when you are in a dangerous situation—hairs on the back of your neck stand up. It tells you when you don't like someone—a gut instinct. Start paying attention to all the many wonderful things your body does for you.

Goddess Workout

Make a list of all the many wonderful things your body does for you.

Write a thank-you letter to your body!

Meditation to Heal a Negative Body Image

Put some relaxing music on your CD player. Close your eyes and do the following meditation:

Imagine you are standing in a beautiful meadow. You are standing on Gaia, the Mother Earth. All around you are beautiful trees, lush flowers, and mossy grass. In the distance you see a clearing. You begin walking toward it now. As you get closer you come to a beautiful waterfall. This is the most gorgeous place you have ever seen. It is like being in a tropical paradise. The air feels humid on your skin and you smell the sweet fragrance of honeysuckle and frangipani. Under your bare feet you feel the damp grass like a soft cushion of the finest velvet.

When you get to the waterfall, you stand underneath it, knowing these are the sacred waters from the body of the Mother. You feel her waters washing away all the pain associated with your bad body image, all the beauty wounds you have received throughout your lifetime. You feel her cleansing waters soothing away the mean things other people have said about your body, any jokes others have made at your expense, any times you have felt shamed, humiliated, or rejected because of your body—all are washed away by the sparkling waterfall.

Washed away are all the times you refused to go out because you didn't want to deal with food or people looking at you. Gone are all the activities and events you have rejected because you were afraid of being rejected yourself. All these are now washed away gently, lovingly, by the sacred waterfalls of Gaia.

You feel the presence of Gaia before you, and then you see her in the clearing, beckoning to you. So you come out of the waterfall and walk slowly toward her. Her face is beaming with so much love for you. You feel so safe and so very secure. You walk toward her and she holds out her arms and embraces you tightly. You fall upon the Earth with her holding you in her lap. She strokes your hair and kisses your face. You feel so very loved and very safe.

She places her hands on your heart and your head and you feel the love of the Great Mother filling you. She pours her love over you in a big magical jug of kindness and comfort. Her love fills you from the top of your head to the bottom of your toes—sparkly pink liquid love radiating through you.

You now feel your body, lush and verdant, abundant as the Earth. Your breasts are like rolling hills, your tummy a round mound, all the dips and crevices, mountains and valleys. You know deep within your being that your body is a perfect expression of the Earth Goddess. Through your body, you are the Goddess made manifest.

You gently bring your attention back to this time, this place, knowing you carry the power of the Goddess within you, and that your relationship with your body will be forever healed.

If you want to get the full benefits of this meditation, record it onto a tape and listen to it every day for thirty days.

Next time you feel like overeating ask yourself: "What am I really hungry for?"

Imagine Gaia holding you in her loving arms, comforting you.

Ask yourself: "What feelings am I trying to suffocate?"

Instead of reaching for food, reach out for the Goddess. Sit down at your computer or with a pen and paper and ask Gaia a question, then write her answer—what you imagine she is saying. When we overeat, we dull our spiritual guidance. Sometimes overeating can be a way of suffocating the messages we are getting.

Ask Gaia: "What messages are you trying to send me?" Write down what she says.

Divine Dieting

When I was a teenager I was forty pounds overweight. For years I struggled with bulimia, compulsive overeating, dieting, and poor body image. My diaries were filled with page after page of me feeling miserable because I was "too fat." I hated the way I looked. I hated the way I felt.

Every Monday was filled with the promise to start a new diet. By Friday my diary was filled with the desperation of feeling out of control around food and feeling miserable because I didn't want to go out and be sociable when I felt fat. I didn't want everyone to see me looking this way and laughing at me behind my back—or worse, to my face.

I know what it is like to cry your eyes out, hanging over the toilet bowl, hating yourself because you've just thrown up for the third time that day. I know what it's like to lie in bed for as late as you can, afraid to get up and have something to eat

334

because you know once you start eating you're not going to be able to stop. I know what it's like to spend every waking hour all day long thinking about food—how much you can eat, how much you can't eat, what you're "allowed" to eat, what you're not. And I know what it is like to let the number on the bathroom scale totally determine how you feel about yourself. Two pounds up is cause for mental torture and overwhelming self-loathing, and two pounds down is reason for great jubilation.

For many years that was my life. My mother put me on my first diet when I was eleven. I can still remember it now, many years later. For breakfast: one cup of skim milk hot chocolate; lunch: one-fourth head of lettuce, one carrot, and one tomato; dinner: one serving of meat, one potato, and another quarter of lettuce, a carrot, and a tomato. That was it. No wonder I was starving! I stayed on that diet solemnly for six weeks. I lost lots of weight. Then one Tuesday night I had my first binge. I stuffed myself with five large sausages, a ton of mashed potatoes, peas, and chocolate cake. "I'll go back on my diet tomorrow," I promised myself. Thus began ten years of dieting, bingeing, and eventually purging.

I tried every diet you could think of. I took diet pills, saw counselors, tried Overeaters Anonymous, and went to an eating disorder clinic. Some things worked temporarily but nothing seemed to stick. By the time I was twenty-two I was burned out, miserable, overweight, and sick and tired of living like that.

That year I made an important decision. I decided I didn't want to spend the rest of my life as a person with an eating disorder. I didn't want to spend the rest of my life obsessed with food and dieting. I wanted to be free. I wanted to live how I imagined a thin person lived—never worrying about food or weight, not spending massive amounts of time reading diet books. I wanted my life back. And I wanted to be strong and healthy and vibrant.

So I threw away all my diet books. I got rid of all the clothes that made me feel frumpy. I bought a good healthy cookbook. I stopped dieting and began making healthy choices on a daily basis, eating foods I enjoyed. Plus I began to exercise every day. Within a year I had lost forty pounds and stopped obsessing about food and weight. But more importantly I felt good about myself.

I'm happy to say that was nearly twenty years ago and I haven't had a weight problem, an eating disorder, or been on a diet since. I have also had two babies, maintained a healthy weight, and continued to exercise on a daily basis. (This is from someone who *dreaded* physical education.)

Anyway, my point is, if you are caught up in the throes of an eating disorder, yo-yo dieting, or bad body image, you don't have to stay there. It is possible to make lasting changes and heal your relationship with food and your body completely. You don't have to understand why you do something in order to change it. Change takes getting up on a daily basis and focusing on what you need to do for that day.

Here are some pointers that helped me:

Banish the Diet Mentality

Clear out all your diet stuff and all the junk food you have lying around. Give away all your diet books. Remember, the more you focus on something, the more power it has. Do you want to spend the rest of your life either on a diet or off one, or would you rather develop lifelong healthy eating habits? The choice is yours.

Find an Eating Style that Empowers You

Every body is different. Your eating style is unique to you. Your body may work more efficiently with a light breakfast, medium lunch, and substantial dinner, or your body might respond better to a hearty breakfast, medium lunch, and light dinner. Perhaps you are the kind of person who works best on five small meals throughout the day. Find out what makes your body respond well.

Eat Only What You Love

Don't waste your time eating foods you hate because they are "good for you." Why eat one single thing you're not crazy about? Instead, find healthy foods you enjoy eating. There are tons of healthy foods to choose from—I am sure you can find at least a few you like.

Make healthier versions of your unhealthy favorites: Bake frozen French fries in the oven, spraying them with Pam, instead of buying French fries from Mac-Donald's. Make chocolate milkshakes by blending milk, frozen yogurt, and chocolate syrup. Dip fresh strawberries, bananas, and apple slices into chocolate syrup for a sweet treat.

Eat Lots of Fruit and Vegetables

What are your favorite fruits? Make sure you buy some the next time you go to the grocery store, or ask your mom to put them on her list. All you need is two pieces of fruit every day and five servings of vegetables to stay healthy.

337

What kind of vegetables do you like?

You can make a great salad quickly with just lettuce, tomato, and a sprinkling of grated cheese.

Drink Lots of Water and Milk

Quit drinking sodas and sugary juices. Limit yourself to one glass every three days if you can't live without them. Drink sparkling water instead of soda. Drink lots of water and you'll speed up your metabolism, flush out toxins, and your skin will love you for it!

Milk is great for building healthy bones, nails, hair, and teeth. Jazz it up by making smoothies with banana and strawberries or other fruit you like.

Eating healthy is just as easy as eating unhealthily.

Exercise Aerobically Every Day

Yep, even if you *hate* exercise. Find an exercise that you enjoy, one that doesn't require much gear or hassle. You could try dancing, rebounding, swimming, walking, cycling, roller-blading, or ice skating. Just put on a CD and dance for twenty minutes in your living room. Get your body moving. Not only will it rev up your metabolism, it will also increase the serotonin levels in your brain so you feel happier.

······································

Goddess Workout

Make a list of your favorite fruits and vegetables.

Make a list of three exercises you are willing to give a try.

Write down what kind of eating style you think will suit your body.

Write down your favorite junk foods. Now come up with some healthy alternatives—this is a chance for you to be really creative.

Remember—goddesses, like girls, come in all shapes and sizes. You don't have to buy into the cultural myth that slim is better or sexier. Be a trailblazer; show people that you are sexy and fabulous. Stick your shoulders back, lift your head up, and walk with pride.

Think of all the different goddesses you have learned about in this book. There is petite Kuan Yin; large, voluptuous Inanna; tall, muscular, athletic Scathach; and curvy Aphrodite. They are all different shapes and they all have amazing magical powers. All of them had challenges that they had to overcome. And they are all beautiful, sexy, and powerful. I can't imagine any one of these goddesses sitting around and crying about her weight or putting her life on hold because she is too fat, too thin, or too whatever—can you?

So remember this: Every time you put your body down, or refuse to do something or be something using your body as an excuse, you are putting the Goddess down. Your body is the physical representation of the Goddess on Earth. You are the Goddess made manifest. Act like one! Which goddess do you think your body most resembles? Find a picture of her and put it on your altar.

Goddess Workout

For the next seven days, commit to being kind to your body. Refuse to say mean things about your body. Refuse to let other people say mean things about your body. And if someone else says something mean about your body to you, stand up for yourself and say, "Don't talk to me like that."

Make a commitment to not say anything mean about anyone else's body for a week, too. If we all did this every day, we would create a place for women to feel safe, no matter what their size.

To put the elements of divine dieting into action, you need to:

1. Create a spiritual blueprint of your ideal self
2. Choose actions and language that support it
3. Call on the Goddess for help every day

Create a Spiritual Blueprint of Your Ideal Self

What do you want to look like? Mentally see an image of yourself standing in front of you. See your body as you would like it to be. See yourself free from any kind of harmful eating behavior. See yourself living a full and active life, participating in all the activities you would like to participate in. See your body as healthy, radiant, and strong. See yourself making healthy choices throughout the day about the kinds of food you will eat. See yourself feeling powerful and in charge. See yourself wearing the kinds of clothes you would love to wear. See yourself happy and confident, feeling great. Put as much energy into this visualization as you can. Remember you are creating an etheric form in the spiritual realm so you can manifest it on the physical plane.

Choose Actions and Language That Support Your Ideal Self

Don't wait until you have lost weight until you start wearing clothes you love or doing activities you'd like to try. Buy yourself a couple of fabulous outfits. There are lots of shops now with great clothes in all sizes. Stop wearing "fat cover-up clothes." These don't truly hide fat and they just make you feel frumpy and miserable, so why wear them? Wear clothes that project the image you want to project. Have at least one great goddess outfit. Force yourself to start doing activities you have been putting off till you lost weight. Participate in life instead of watching life go by while you go on a diet.

Choose actions that support the ideal image you have of yourself.

Call on the Goddess Every Day for Help

See the Goddess helping you reach your desired weight and healing your relationship with food. Remember, the Goddess can do anything and even if it feels really overwhelming to you to eat healthy and feel great, it is certainly not overwhelming for her. So just put it all in her hands and expect help.

Pray:

Dearest Gaia

I ask you to heal my relationship with food today

Help me to cherish my body

To treat it lovingly and with respect

Help me to choose healthy foods to eat

To exercise today

And to feel great about myself!

Gaia's Glamour

- Bold, bright colors that invoke a summer's day awash with flowers, brilliance, and fertility, like hot pink, lime green, canary yellow, and orange
- Floral dresses
- Long chiffon skirts
- Short baby tees in any of the above colors
- Gold hoop earrings
- Fuchsia glossy lipstick

Makeup

Wash your face and apply a sun bronzer to your skin. Line your eyes with forest green eyeliner and apply sky blue eye cream to your eyelids. Accentuate with lots of black mascara. Apply peach cream blush to your cheeks and a raspberry lipstick to your lips. Dab gold glitter above your cheekbones and across your shoulder bones.

Clothing

Choose colors that represent the abundance of the Earth. Anything with a floral print or even a fruit print is good. Alternatively you can choose clothes in the color of the Earth like rich browns, greens, or golds. Wear clothes that show off your body. The Earth is Gaia's body, and your body is a manifestation of the Goddess.

Wear fresh flowers in your hair or sprinkle flower petals in your hair. Wear flower necklaces, daisy chains, or sparkly gold bracelets.

Ceremony

Get dressed up in your Gaia gear. Have some fresh floral perfume handy.

Say a prayer:

Dearest Gaia

Please be with me now

Let me feel your loving presence

And so it is

Amen

Close your eyes and imagine you are an ancient priestess who trained at the Greek temples and spent her life devoted to the Goddess. Take the perfume into your hands and put some on your index finger.

Now anoint your feet. Say: "Blessed are your feet, for they walk in the ways of the Goddess."

Next anoint your knees, saying: "Blessed are your knees, which kneel at her holy altar."

Anoint your womb: "Blessed be your womb from which all life proceeds."

Anoint your breasts: "Blessed be your breasts that sustain sacred life."

Then your lips: "Blessed be your lips that speak the hallowed words."

Finally anoint your forehead and say: "You are goddess, (your name)."

Now go out into the world as Gaia the earth goddess, and spread your abundance everywhere!

Gaia's Tasks for You

- Write a letter to an editor of a women's magazine that promotes a wide variety of models in all shapes and sizes, or one that has good body image articles. Commend them for their empowering work. Alternatively you can write a letter to the editor of a magazine that you feel disempowers women and tell them you don't like their limited stance.

- Make a clay goddess figurine of yourself as a goddess, modeling on your own body shape. Give her a goddess name.

- Spend one day this week as Gaia the earth goddess. Be kind and giving, knowing there is plenty more where whatever you give comes from. You are lush and verdant like the Earth. You are perfectly in rhythm with your body. How does it feel to be the Earth Goddess? Write about it in your goddess diary.

*C*elebrate your body!

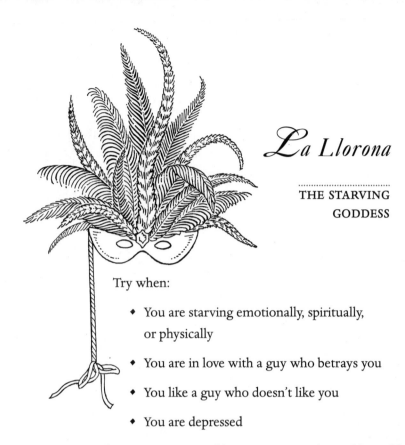

La Llorona

Try when:

- You are starving emotionally, spiritually, or physically

- You are in love with a guy who betrays you

- You like a guy who doesn't like you

- You are depressed

La Llorona (pronounced *la-your-own-a*) is the goddess of broken hearts. She is the weeping woman of the American Southwest who walks along the Rio Grande calling out for her lost children.

La Llorona drowned her dreams for the love of a man. She knows the madness of losing your identity in love, having your dreams shattered and then destroying yourself and your world in a moment of craziness born of inconsolable grief. She knows what it is like to come to your senses and have to face the horror of what you have done.

La Llorona begs you to learn from her story rather than follow her example. Her message is a warning: "Do not follow where I have walked. Cherish your dreams and take responsibility to make them beautiful. Let them live, as if your life depends upon it—for indeed it does."

La Llorona's Story

The weeping woman of the Southwest

Once upon a time, a long, long time ago, there lived a beautiful young girl named Maria. She had long hair as dark as a raven, olive skin that shone like a finely polished apple, and large black eyes. The village people where she lived thought she was the most beautiful girl in the world, and whenever Maria walked by they would whisper behind their hands, "Surely she becomes more beautiful with each passing day."

As she grew older her beauty increased. Many of the young men in her village longed to date her, but Maria had set her sights on something more. She was not content to stay poor and live a life of hardship in her little village where people never amounted to much. She wanted more from her life. She wanted to see what the world could offer her. She had dreams—passionate dreams of living a life of luxury in a beautiful home surrounded by art and music, with little children running around her feet, a handsome man at her side, dinner parties and intellectual conversation. Maria wanted to make something of her life. She yearned to make art, to write poetry, to converse long into the night about something more than the local village gossip.

One day a dashing ranchero rode into Maria's village. He was finely dressed and could ride just like a Comanche. Maria soon learned he was the son of a wealthy rancher. He was so rich that if one of the horses he rode grew too tame for his liking, he would give it away. Then he would go rope another wild horse from the plains. Maria had never seen someone so worldly with so much money and so much finesse. Plus he was so handsome, with his long dark hair and piercing brown eyes. Sometimes he would sit outside the casa where he was staying and play his guitar, singing hauntingly beautiful songs of places far away. Maria could see the places in her imagination and indeed it seemed as if she were in another world whenever she was near him.

He was the most beautiful man Maria had ever laid eyes on. Whenever she looked at him she felt her heart burst open with much joy and happiness. He came from far away, from a wealthy family, while she lived in a tiny cottage with dirt for a floor and barely enough money to put food on the table. He knew so much about the world and talked of things she had never heard of, while her conversations were limited to what went on in the village around her. Hungrily, Maria listened to every word she could catch him saying, for through him she could catch a glimpse of far-off places.

So whenever she could take a break from her daily chores, Maria would stop and linger by the stoop where he sat playing his guitar. It wasn't long before the ranchero noticed her, of course, for her beauty was beguiling. But it was her soul that captured him, for he saw in Maria a deep longing, a hunger for life that matched his own. So he began singing songs especially for her, and brought her gifts from the city after each visit: a tiny paint box and paper so she could paint her dreams, a book of poetry wrapped in a brown leather case, seashells and minuscule bottles filled with seawater.

And before long it was more than their dreams and conversations that the two were sharing. They became lovers and the ranchero bought a little cottage on the edge of the village that they moved into. Maria was so happy; she had never been happier in all her life, happy to be loved by a beautiful man, to be able to paint and read and feed her soul. Each day was an opportunity to see more beauty and feel more love, and when she became pregnant with his child she felt she carried the soul of divine love itself within her.

For several years they lived like this, the ranchero and Maria, producing two children. At times the ranchero would go back to the city and stay for months at a time to visit his family. He never took Maria or their children with him, and Maria never asked why. But at night when he was gone she would stare out at the stars and wonder if perhaps he was ashamed of her. When he returned, he would be so full of love for her that all her doubts were washed away. He would come back bearing gifts for her and the children and the house would be filled with love and laughter, and Maria would wonder why she had ever doubted him in the first place.

Then one time after these visits to his family the ranchero returned and Maria felt a change in him. He seemed distant from her; he did not reach out to touch her quite as much, and he spent more time going for long rides in the desert alone. He did not seem to pay as much attention to the children either. Indeed, he seemed preoccupied in his own little world. So Maria questioned him about it.

345

At first he denied that anything was wrong. But then finally he burst out, "Oh, Maria, I am so sorry. I am bequeathed to another woman. My family has arranged a marriage for me and if I do not marry I will lose everything—all my wealth, my title, everything."

"But you will not lose me," stated Maria. "You will not lose our family."

"You do not understand, Maria," he hurled at her. "I still love you, but I am no longer in love with you. I am in love with someone else."

"No!" Maria snapped. "It is *you* who do not understand. You already have a family."

"We can still be friends, Maria," he tried.

"Friends?" Maria screamed. "Friends, you think I want to be friends with someone who treats me like this? What makes you think I would want to be your friend?"

"Maria—" he began.

But Maria was consumed with hurt. She felt her heart breaking. The pain was overwhelming—gone were her dreams of a life spent loving this man, gone were her dreams of a better life for herself.

"I am just a silly foolish girl, with silly foolish dreams," she cried. "Why would I believe someone as wonderful as you could love me?"

"Maria—"

She grabbed her paint box, her paintings, her fine leather-bound books and tore them apart, hurling the shreds at the floor. Then she grabbed her two small children and, crying, stumbled out of the house.

The ranchero did not know what to do. "She will get over it," he thought. "Let her go, let her cry, then she will be okay."

But Maria was not okay. Her grief overwhelmed her. As passionate as her love was, so, too, was the hurt. Wailing, she stumbled down to the river, a child in each arm, and when she got there she fell to the ground. She could see no future, she could see no past. All she could see was more pain. "Oh, my poor children," she wept. "May you not have to suffer as I have had to suffer." And she threw the children into the river and let the rushing water carry them away.

As their little bodies disappeared on the current, Maria realized what she had done. "Oh, dear god!" she cried. She ran down the riverbank reaching out her arms to them, screaming their names over and over, but they were long gone.

The next morning a traveler found Maria dead by the side of the river, her arms outstretched toward the water. He picked her up and took her back to the village where she was buried in a long white gown in the village cemetery.

But that night the villagers heard a woman wailing, "Where are my children? Where are my children?" And they peeked out their windows and saw a ghostly woman as thin as a skeleton, wearing a long white gown, pacing up and down the riverbank with her arms outstretched.

347

On many a dark night, they heard her cry for her children and saw her floating above the river. So they no longer talked about her as Maria. Instead they named her La Llorona, the weeping woman. And by that name she is known today. Children are warned not to go out after dark, for La Llorona in her grief might snatch them and never return them.

The Message of La Llorona

La Llorona is the Mexican goddess of the starving soul. She is the weeping woman who cries in the night for the two small children she drowned for the love of a man. She is the part of ourselves who abandons a piece of our souls when we love those who do not love us back.

La Llorona is the tragic tale of unrequited love. La Llorona is a poor peasant girl who gives her heart to a rich boyfriend. She bears him two sons and oh, she is *so* happy, she is *sooo* in love with him, surely one day he will see how wonderful she is and marry her. He is so handsome, intelligent, wealthy, and dashing. He has all the confidence in the world and when she is with him her own world feels a little more magical and a little more like the impossible is possible.

I love this bittersweet love story for two reasons. One because for many years I spent my life living like La Llorona, obsessing about some guy, dating those who did not deserve my love and certainly did not return it. I threw away my talents, my dreams, my desires, my money, my time, my attention, and my self-worth, and poured it all into my relationships in the hopes that some day this boy would "wake up" and love me, too.

What I really should have been doing was building a strong relationship with myself, and feeding my own dreams.

How many times have you drowned your talents, your creativity, your yearnings, and your inner dreams for the love of another? Many women have lived the story of La Llorona—some literally drown their children, like Susan Smith. Some drown their souls. Whatever your choices, don't do it. It is simply not worth it.

The second reason I love this story is because it hails from the Southwest, where I live. Sometimes I walk along the Rio Grande listening, listening for the wails of grief from La Llorona.

Goddess Workout

Write about a time when you were betrayed by love. What happened? How did you cope with the pain?

Has there ever been a time when you have put your dreams on hold, buried a part of yourself, or stopped expressing your talents because of your love for another?

Have you ever dated someone who made you feel belittled in some way? If so, in what ways?

Lessons of the Dark Goddess

La Llorona is a dark goddess. The lessons of this goddess are profound and almost unbearably painful, but the pain is a portal into greater wisdom and compassion. Be like Scathach and wear your scars with pride. Your scars do not define you. The scars of love do not define you. Your life is like a large beautiful tapestry with many colors woven into it. When painful events occur, they become woven into the overall beauty of the tapestry, adding depths and dimensions that were not there previously. Your life as a whole can still be beautiful, even in the midst of great inner turmoil.

From inner pain you learn strength, from fear comes compassion, and from turmoil comes transformation.

How to Heal a Broken Heart

Have you ever been betrayed by love? Have you ever felt pain so overwhelming there seemed to be no escape from it? If that is where you are at today, then try the following:

Turn It Over to the Goddess

There is nothing the Goddess cannot heal. When your pain is so great it feels as if your heart will literally break, light a candle and talk to the Goddess. Call upon La Llorona, who certainly understands the power of grieving love's losses. Pray to La Llorona:

Dear Goddess

Please come to me now

My heart is hurting

Pour your loving balm

Into my heart

Take my pain

And make me whole again

When your heart breaks, you may wonder if it will ever heal again. It's important to know that healing begins the moment wounding takes place. When you cut your finger, your body immediately begins the healing process necessary to repair the wound. So it is with emotional healing.

Broken hearts mend stronger than hearts that have never been broken, just as broken bones mend stronger than bones that have never been broken. Scar tissue is stronger than regular skin tissue.

When hearts break, they break open so they can contain more love. When it feels like you are shattering inside, you are breaking open so new life can form and grow. Just remember to talk to the Goddess because she will guide you through your grief and sorrow. You are not alone.

Make a Bag of Sorrows

Get a plain paper bag and write on it with a marker "Bag of Sorrows." This is where you are going to store all the things that make you unhappy. Each day write down what made you unhappy that day. Write down all the things that hurt about the betrayal, all the reasons why "no man will ever love you again." Write down all the things you feel powerless over. Put the pieces of paper into your bag of sorrows.

Whenever an unhappy thought comes up, write it down and put it in your bag of sorrows. At the end of a month, burn your bag of sorrows at the dark of the moon.

Call on the Power of Your Ancestors

Call on your ancestors to help you. They can help you in a multitude of ways, like providing you comfort and lending you strength. Your ancient ancestors probably have all kinds of skills that can help you. They may have been warriors or priestesses or any number of wonderful things. So call on your ancestors to empower you with their strengths at this time.

Use Your Goddess Power to Banish the Pain and the Bad Memories

Part of being a goddess-in-training is learning how to banish. As a goddess girl you have the power to banish and manifest whatever you need. To banish the pain, you simply have to stop paying it so much attention. I know this is hard when you have been hurt, but it is not impossible. The Goddess once told me when I felt as if I was literally dying of a broken heart, "You must use your magic to make the bad stuff go away."

How do you do this? By making a conscious choice not to hang out in the land of pain and suffering. This means when the pain comes up you must tell yourself, "I can get through this, I can do hard things, the Goddess is with me, helping me now."

When a bad memory comes to mind, you say, "Okay, this is what I am feeling now but it is not what I want to be experiencing. Now I would rather experience peace of mind, hope, and joy." Then think of something wonderful happening to you in the near future.

....

Goddess Workout

Write down three wonderful things you would like to experience in the future.

1.

2.

3.

Whenever a painful memory emerges, deliberately replace it with one of the things on your list. Do this as many times as necessary during the day. We are literally washing your brain out!

Keen Your Grief and Rage

Keening is a sacred magical practice from both the Maori tradition and the Celtic tradition. In times of great sorrow women would keen, which is a loud piercing wail of grief from the pits of their stomachs. When my mother died, I learned to keen from two of my Maori elders. Whenever I am in a place of great grief, the Goddess reminds me to keen. Keening is a very powerful way to release hurt, anger, and pain.

How to Keen

1. Find a quiet place where no one will hear you. You can use your car, if necessary.

2. Close your eyes.

3. Tune into all the hurt and pain and anger.

4. Imagine two priestesses standing on either side of you, holding your arms to give you support.

5. Let out a loud wail from the base of your belly.

6. Do this as many times as necessary, until you feel the pain start to subside.

See the Goddess Healing You

Close your eyes, lie down, and imagine the Goddess holding you in her arms. She is rocking you like she would a child. Imagine her as your kind, loving mother. Once when I was hurting from a broken heart, the Goddess came to me and told me to think of her quite literally as my mother. My mother was already dead and the Goddess told me that whenever I had a problem or a heartache to go to her just as I would want to go to a regular mother. She has held me in her arms all night long to soothe me after a painful experience.

So imagine the Goddess holding you in her arms, wrapped lovingly around you. She places her healing hands on your heart and fills it with love. She places her hands across your forehead and soothes your mind. She makes all things new again. She gives you hope.

Take Small Steps to Begin Feeding Your Soul

What do you love to do? In times of grief it is important to take good care of yourself. This means making sure you get enough rest, get some exercise, and eat properly. Often simple things can feel overwhelming if you are sad or depressed. Do them anyway. There have been days when I have had to force myself to get out of bed, get dressed, and go for a walk. Sometimes it seems even more unfair when the people whom you feel have caused you pain seem to be getting on with their lives without any problem. Don't worry about them, worry about you! Your suffering only hurts you.

This is a great time to do nice things for yourself. Get involved in something creative, learn a new hobby, write poetry, make a photo collage. Express yourself in some way. Some of my most poignant poems have come from times of great grief.

Light a Candle

This is a good way to rekindle the light spark within you. Light a candle and talk to the Goddess. Let this candle symbolize your passion, your desires. Let it flame your soul back to life. Each day spend ten minutes focusing on the flame of the candle. Just meditate by watching the flame. See the Goddess walking ahead of you one step at a time, holding your arm to propel you forward. See her holding a candle in front of you to illuminate your path. Know that you do not need to know the answer to every question and that you will always be divinely guided and protected.

Write Down All the Things You Could Gain
from This Happening

This is a way to look for gold in a pile of dirt. You may have more free time, you may have learned how to love yourself in the face of adversity, or you may have learned a lot about forgiveness and compassion. The most heartbreaking experience I ever went through taught me a lot about forgiveness and my ability to love in the midst of chaos. I also discovered what wonderful friends I had. They were incredibly supportive. Would I rather not have experienced the heartache? Yes, of course, but knowing there were some positive outcomes helped me cope with it, too. In every tragedy there are silver linings. Catastrophes can bring out the best in people. What have you learned from the situation?

Stop Asking Why It Happened

Asking why bad things happen inevitably trips you up. There is no logical, rational explanation for betrayal. "Shit happens." This does not excuse another's bad behavior, but you may never understand why it happened and that is okay. Trying to get the person who hurt you to give you a "reasonable" explanation of why they did it is a waste of time. You will probably never be satisfied with what they say. Instead of focusing on things you can't change, move your attention to things you can.

Remember:

- Although grieving takes time, the idea is to get out of the pain as quickly as possible—that means not looking back.

- Bad stuff always seems to happen at the worst possible time: the holidays, Christmas, your birthday, Valentine's Day.

- When you put the past in front of you, you create a roadblock for the future.

- You will not only survive this, but thrive.

- Scar tissue is stronger than regular skin tissue.

- When a bone breaks it heals stronger than it was before.

- Your heart is the strongest muscle in your entire body— it can heal and it will heal.

You have many choices:

- What you want to do today.

- How you want to make your life better.

- What kind of relationship you want to be in.

One day you will look back on the hard times and see they were defining moments in your life. Time heals not because it makes heartbreaking experiences go away but because it gives us a different perspective of the situation. We can look back from a distance and see how far we have come, the choices we have made, how we have learned, and how life has led us in a different direction. Just like an artist must step back from her painting while she is working on it to see the overall expression from the finer details so, too, must you be like an artist and step back at various stages of your life to see how all the parts fit together.

I believe life is very wise. Sometimes things that happen that seem just absolutely intolerable at the time can lead us into a whole different direction for our lives. These are our defining moments. Remember when I said that I would rather not have experienced the heartache? Well, now I'm not so sure that is completely true. Yes, heartache sucks and I would rather not have to feel it. But there is a certain beauty in times of great sorrow and looking back I can see how the painful events of my life have transformed me; they have deepened my soul, stretched my understanding of others, and expanded my capacity for love, compassion, and empathy. How can I help another soul through a dark time if I have never experienced my own times of despair? Holding the light of hope for another who is hurting and being able to say "you will get through this" with absolute conviction because you have gotten through it yourself at one time is such a beautiful gift to be able to give.

La Llorona's Glamour

- Crimson lipstick

- Peasant blouse

- Long full skirt

- Mexican skirt with embroidered flowers around the hem

- Silver bangles, turquoise jewelry

- Leather sandals

- Black lacy shawl

La Llorona was very glamorous. That was one of the things that attracted her lover to her. You see, you don't have to be rich to have glamour. True glamour is an inward quality, not an outward possession. La Llorona carried herself with grace and self-possession, aware of her heavy sensuality that attracted others to her.

Makeup

La Llorona's makeup is earth-toned colors for the eyes and cheeks, and red lipstick for the lips. Line your eyes with black eyeliner. Then apply a rich brown eye shadow to your eyelids all the way above the crease. You can apply a light gold eye shadow to your brow bone, too. Next apply a liquid black eyeliner to your upper lids, all the way from the inner corner of the eye to the outer corner, ending with a slight sweep upwards. Use lots of dark mascara to make your lashes thick.

Color your eyebrows in a shade darker than your normal coloring with a brow pencil.

Apply gold highlighter to your cheeks and forehead.

Apply a red lipstick to your lips with a lip brush.

Clothing

Try a full skirt with a little white T-shirt and sandals. Dress it up with a silver belt, hoop earrings, and silver and turquoise jewelry. Add a shawl either tied around your waist or draped around your shoulders, and you are ready to go. A large flower pinned in your hair or at your waist is a great accessory.

Ceremony

This ceremony is for calling your soul back to you. Part of La Llorona's lesson was losing her soul and searching for it again. When you go through a traumatic loss, be it a rejection, a betrayal, a death, or any kind of loss, part of your soul can stay in the loss. This may lead to severe depression, anxiety, addictive behavior, or feelings of hopelessness and apathy. You may feel off-center, as if your life no longer has any meaning. You may push aside your dreams and just want to curl up on the couch doing nothing. This is a great time to do soul retrieval. This is where you travel into the spirit world and call the lost parts of your soul back to your physical body.

So for this ceremony we are going to travel into the spirit world with the help of La Llorona and bring the parts of your soul that you have lost back to you.

To begin your journey, you need two things: a quiet place where you can relax, like your bedroom, and a piece of music that helps you to move into a deep meditative state. It is best to use instrumental music, not music with words, unless it is a chanting tape. There are tapes that are made especially for traveling into the spirit world, such as Michael Harner's tapes for the shamanic journey or Robert Gass's tapes with chants on them.

Get dressed in your La Llorona costume.

Put your music on and cast a magic circle by standing in the east and closing your eyes. Hold your right arm out in front of you with your index finger pointed straight out. If you are left-handed, use your left hand. Visualize a blue flame coming from your index finger the color of a gas pilot light. Now walk around in a circle, imagining the blue flame extending from your finger, until you have made a complete circle.

357

Hold both your arms above your head, palms together and fingers pointing upwards. Invoke La Llorona by praying:

La Llorona

Goddess of grieving

You know the heartache of lost love

You know the sadness of losing your dreams

You know well the feelings of hopelessness and depression

That can come in times of great sorrow

Come to me now, dear Goddess

To help me find my soul center again

Lie down on the floor and close your eyes. Imagine La Llorona is with you. Together you are going to go on a journey. La Llorona takes you by the hand and pulls you up off the floor. In your imagination, you go out through your front door, and she pulls you up into the sky. Together you fly for several minutes until she brings you to a riverbank. You stand by the river with her. The current is strong and flowing fast beside you.

La Llorona calls out for your lost soul. You hear her saying your name over and over, calling out for your lost soul to return back to you. She calls to the river for help, she calls to the moon and the sun and the stars. She calls to your ancestors.

"Help (your name) remember her power. Bring her power back to her now!" she says.

Pretty soon you see the last fragments of your soul flying toward you. La Llorona reaches out and clasps them in her hands. She holds them to her heart for several moments. Then she gently holds them in her hands and blows them into your body, all the way from your head down to your toes. You feel a jolt of power enter you.

La Llorona beckons you to sit down by the river. She sits across from you and holds your hands. "My dear child," she says, "many are the loves you will have in your life and many are the loves you will lose. You will see all the faces of love across the tapestry of your life. Just remember that you are always rooted in spiritual soil. Your soul's sustenance comes from no one person but rather from Spirit itself. Though the channels of love may change, the source will not. Just as this river is fed by one source, so too is your heart fed by the one divine source.

"The way to heal hurt is to focus on love until there is no room for the hurt anymore."

You stay with La Llorona for a few more minutes, asking her whatever questions you wish. When you are ready, you come back to this time and this place.

La Llorona's Tasks for You

+ Go out into the world as La Llorona for a day. How does it feel to be her? Write your experience in your goddess diary.

+ Write a love poem.

+ Take a walk by a river and sit under a tree and draw a picture or read a book. Have a picnic and talk to La Llorona.

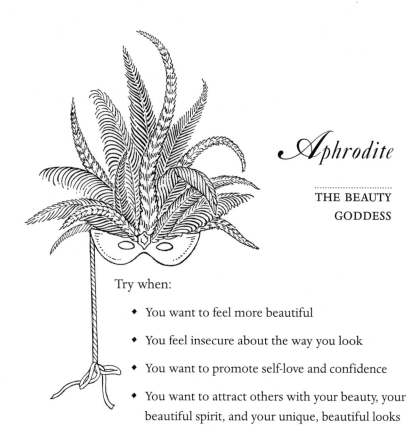

Aphrodite

THE BEAUTY GODDESS

Try when:

- ◆ You want to feel more beautiful

- ◆ You feel insecure about the way you look

- ◆ You want to promote self-love and confidence

- ◆ You want to attract others with your beauty, your beautiful spirit, and your unique, beautiful looks

Aphrodite (pronounced *a-fro-die-tee*) is the goddess of love, beauty, and wisdom. She always has tons of guys falling all over her. She is radiantly beautiful and enchanting. When Cleopatra wanted to get Mark Antony to fall in love with her, she dressed up as Aphrodite and sailed into Antony's port in a golden ship with billowing purple sails. Cleopatra knew the power of using her imagination, spirituality, and physical props to invoke a goddess. She also knew the power of Aphrodite to attract love and beauty.

Aphrodite is so beautiful men and gods fall instantly in love with her. She is the golden goddess and everywhere she walks men and women bask in the golden glow of her love. She exudes beauty, love, and wisdom like a walking sun, so all who come across her are warmed by her sunny nature.

Her hair is long and golden and lights up the sky like a golden halo. Her eyes are azure blue and sprinkle love on those she gazes at. Her body is lush and fertile like a summer's tree bursting with fruit. Her voice is as sweet as honey dripping off buttered toast.

In her myths, Aphrodite faced many trials. She was married to Hephaestus, the Greek god of the forge. Hephaestus was crippled, and he made many items of great beauty, which was one of the reasons Aphrodite was attracted to him. However, Aphrodite had many lovers, which often got her into trouble. She danced with Dionysus, the god of love and ecstasy, who had a reputation for making girls crazy; she seduced Ares and got caught in a trap set for her by the other gods.

She initiated Psyche into her own goddess power by giving her seemingly impossible tasks to complete. Aphrodite will make you aware of the power of beauty and how you can create it at will. She will initiate you into your own goddess power by giving you the knowledge that you can complete impossible tasks through action, too.

Aphrodite's Story

How Aphrodite initiated Psyche

Now it has been said that I was jealous of Psyche because she was a mortal who was incredibly beautiful. However, let it be known that that is hogwash, as I am the golden goddess of beauty and it is my divine beauty I bestow on mortals. Therefore, what have I to be jealous of? How well it pleases me to behold the beauty of another.

However, beauty without wisdom is a dangerous quality. It leaves you vulnerable to those who would use you, misuse you, or abuse you simply for your beauty. And that is what it was with Psyche. She had beauty but no wisdom. And because she was pregnant with my grandchild, I decided to train her, to awaken her own goddess power. For what good is it if I simply lend her mine whenever she is in difficulty? That way, she would have gained nothing.

It all began when my son Eros arranged for Psyche to be brought to his castle. Psyche was unaware of what was happening. All she knew was that she had been transported to the most beautiful palace in the entire universe.

Each night she would go to bed in her magnificent bedroom and be met by a strange man who would make love with her all night long. However, she never saw his face. And indeed this mysterious lover asked Psyche to swear never to attempt to see him, to which she willingly agreed.

Now this arrangement went on for many months. Psyche played happily throughout the castle during the day, never lacking for anything. As darkness fell she was joined by her husband. Although she could not see him, she knew him by his touch, by his smell, his laughter, his taste, and the very essence of his being. Psyche loved him dearly.

However, her girlfriends thought this arrangement rather strange.

"Perhaps he is ugly," they suggested. "Perhaps he has the face of an imbecile or is hideously disfigured."

"I don't care," retorted Psyche. "He is beauty itself to me."

But the girls were relentless in their taunting. They teased Psyche so much that one night, forgetting her promise, she rose from her marriage bed and lit a candle to gaze upon the face of her beloved. This was no ugly monster, but the most beautiful face she had ever laid eyes on. It was the face of Eros—none other than my mischievous son!

A drop of scalding wax fell upon the god's cheek. He jumped from the bed, scolding Psyche for her lack of faith.

"Could you not trust me?" he demanded. "I have given you everything. Now you have broken your vow and I must go until you are worthy of my love." With that he vanished into thin air, taking the castle with him. Poor Psyche was left alone, perched on a rock with only her grief for company.

She was like that when I found her. She pleaded for my help to locate Eros. I agreed, provided she completed four tasks for me first. Here, then, are the tasks I gave her.

1. Sorting the Seeds

I led Psyche into a room that contained an enormous mountain of seeds all jumbled together. There was corn, barley, lentils, millet, poppy seeds, and beans.

"Psyche," I told her, "you must sort each seed into a pile of its like kind before the sun sets."

By doing this I was teaching her how to be discerning, to sort the "good" seeds from the "bad." Discernment is an important step in using your goddess power, as is a keen eye and attention to detail. By completing this task, along with the help of some friendly ants, Psyche learned to trust the power of her spiritual sight and to practice wise judgment.

2. Acquiring Some Golden Fleece

Next I ordered her to get some golden fleece from the rams of the sun. These rams are huge vicious beasts. If Psyche went into their midst she would surely be smashed to smithereens.

Psyche waited until dark when the rams lay down to rest. As they lay sleeping, she picked several strands of fleece, which she promptly brought to me.

"Well done, Psyche," I praised. "You have learned the art of waiting and observing to know what you are up against. You have learned to focus your energies before tackling a difficult task. You are learning to trust your intuition and act with divine guidance instead of blundering in blindly and causing yourself to be vulnerable to danger."

3. Filling the Flask with Magic Water

Now I gave Psyche a tiny crystal flask and told her: "You must fill this flask from the stream over yonder."

"But there are dragons there guarding it," wept Psyche. "And how am I supposed to get to it? For it runs as high as the tallest mountain and as low as the middle of the Earth itself."

"Psyche, just DO IT!" I admonished.

Psyche waited until an eagle came to aid her, and together they flew above the dragons and above the stream, swooping down to retrieve some of the magic water.

"Good job, Psyche," I said. "You have learned to rise above your problems and your emotions, and see solutions from a different perspective, a spiritual perspective. And you have learned that there are many goddess helpers to assist you on your path at all times."

4. *Journey to the Underworld*

Now, for the most terrifying task of all, I sent Psyche to the underworld, with a small box to be filled with beauty ointment from Persephone.

The underworld is a scary place, filled with the most horrifying sights you can imagine. Hanging skeletons, leering monsters, all kinds of hideous visions. But the worst thing about it is there you come face-to-face with your own worst fear. Some people who enter into its murky depths never return.

I gave Psyche a condition to this task. "You will see many lost souls wandering around down there," I warned. "But under no condition are you at liberty to help them. Three times you must refuse to help another. If you give in, all will be lost and you will stay down there forever!"

In this way Psyche learned to face her worst fears and her deepest pain, and see the strength that is gained from such a journey. She learned to harden her heart to the pleas of others who would distract her from her path. Now at last Psyche had learned how to use her own goddess power, and no one could ever take it from her again. She was, of course, reunited with Eros as his equal, and they lived happily together for many years.

How to Create Beauty In Every Area of Your Life

Our society holds many myths about beauty. As girls we grow up hearing stories about beautiful princesses who get attacked by ugly stepmothers, then saved by handsome princes. As teenagers we read magazines that tell us how to become beautiful by following certain "rules." Here are some of the rules that were on the cover of this month's magazines:

- ◆ Try our quick do-it-yourself makeover tricks

- ◆ Put your bikini body on ice: fat busters that work

These magazines often follow up with articles on how to make a boy fall in love with you: "The secret language of guys—50 clues he is crazy about you." Then we learn beauty and boys go hand in hand.

Who makes up these myths? The media? Our culture? It doesn't really matter except that many of us grow up with a distorted idea of what beauty is and how to attain it. Here are some of the myths we learn about beauty:

- Beautiful people are born beautiful

- Beauty is determined by your size, shape, age, or a combination of physical factors

- Beauty must be validated in order to count

In other words, unless someone else tells you that you are beautiful, you are not. You can't possibly call yourself beautiful unless you fit the criteria of our society. Even then you are not supposed to think of yourself as beautiful because that would be vain. What a load of rubbish!

So if we grow up with a false or limited definition of what beautiful is, how do we create our own? According to my dictionary, *beauty* means the quality that gives pleasure to the sight or aesthetic pleasure in general. Aesthetic includes all five senses so another definition of beauty could be a quality that gives the senses pleasure.

"Beautify" means to make beautiful, grace, or adorn, and "beatify" means to make blessed or happy. Grace means an easy elegance in the form of manners and also divine influence. So with these definitions in tow, we can begin to expand our understanding of beauty as a quality that is spiritual and emotional—a quality which goes way beyond mere physical dimensions.

If we want to become beautiful, we need to focus on the spiritual and emotional aspects of beauty as much as improving our physical appearance. When you grow spiritually and emotionally, your physical appearance will change, too. When you stop trying to live up to outer ideals or expectations and look within to find the answers of how you wish to live and look, then beauty is suddenly attainable, instead of being an elusive quality that is always just out of reach, which no amount of primping, preening, or products can produce.

Beauty, according to the mystic Kahlil Gibran, is "a heart inflamed and a soul enchanted." What are the things which inflame your heart and enchant your soul? Write them down in your goddess journal. What are you passionate about? Begin to focus on the things that enchant your soul and ignite your passion. Create beauty in the way you speak, the way you act, and the things that you do. Bring beauty into all areas of your life. A flower here, a kind word there, a smile at the stranger on the street . . . pretty soon you will find that beauty has found you. Let Beauty be your guide. If you look into the mirror and only see flaws, you need to call Beauty into your life. Call on Aphrodite, the goddess of beauty, for help.

367

Beauty is the radiance of your soul's light shining forth. When you live in accordance with your inner spirit and connect to the spirit of the Goddess, the beauty of divinity illuminates you from within. You do not need to rely on your own resources to be beautiful. You can invoke the beauty of the universe, the beauty of the Goddess, the beauty of the stars, the sun, and the moon to shine through you.

Beauty is your birthright. Claim it now!

Meditation to Increase Your Beauty

This is a walking meditation so you will need to wear comfortable shoes—or better yet go barefoot. Go for a twenty-minute walk, observing beauty wherever you go. Notice the beauty that is all around you. If you can't see any, then *look harder.* See the beauty of the sky, the beauty of the weather, the beauty of the trees, the beauty of people on the streets, the beauty of storefronts. Use all your senses. See what smells you come across. Take a moment to touch things— pick up a stone or dance your fingertips across a glass window. Do what delights you. Honor the beauty in the universe. Honor the beauty of this day. Honor the beauty that is within you.

When you invite Beauty into your heart, she herself will be your guide . . .

Another Meditation to Increase Your Beauty

Every night for one month gaze at the moon for ten minutes. You need to do this for a full month so you go through the entire moon cycle. The moon is magnetic and if you stand under her gentle gaze, you will become magnetized, too. She will make you more luminous, more alluring. You can talk to the moon while you do this. Tell her how you desire to be more attractive. Let her bathe you with her silvery rays. Don't be surprised if she talks back to you!

Goddess Workout

Get a roll of toilet paper and a pen.

Write down on each piece of paper one reason why you can't be beautiful. You know the "reasons." You have probably been telling yourself them for a long time. Or maybe someone else has told you. Or perhaps you've gotten the messages from the media, women's magazines, films, or music, the messages that say "Beauty looks like this, and it's not YOU!"

Anyway, write down all the reasons why you can't be beautiful right now, today.

Your list might look something like this:

I'm too fat

I'm too thin

My nose is too big

I have skinny knees

Joey says I'm ugly

My skin is bad

Keep writing until you have exhausted every single reason you can think of.

Now take the scraps of toilet paper and flush them down the toilet. That is where those reasons belong. They are crap! You are beautiful, right now, this minute. So just flush all that crap away, down the toilet where it belongs. Then have a quick shower to wash off any of the residue from those thought forms.

Now you are going to begin affirming your beauty.

Prayer for Beauty

Open my heart, O Goddess

Open my heart to the beauty of my life

The beauty of my love

The beauty of my spirit

Open my heart, O Goddess

To the beauty of this day

The beauty of the sun

The beauty of the stars

The beauty of the trees

Open my heart, O Goddess

To the beauty of my relationships

The beauty of my friends

The beauty of my loved ones

Open my heart, O Goddess

To the beauty of my hair

The beauty of my toes

The beauty of my heart

The beauty of my thighs

The beauty of my sight

The beauty of my voice

The beauty of my breath

The beauty of my skin

The beauty of my touch

The beauty of my nose

The beauty of my tummy

The beauty of my lungs

Open my heart, O Goddess

To the beauty that is ME

Affirmations for Beauty

- I invoke the spirit of beauty

- I invite beauty into all areas of my life

- Beauty herself will guide me to my true beauty

- Every day I become more and more beautiful

- I am a work of art in progress

- The beauty of the Goddess radiates through me

- I weave beauty around me

Magical Makeup: Using Makeup as a Magical Tool

Makeup is magical. With makeup you can create an illusion of how you wish to appear. Today there is an endless variety of makeup supplies to choose from. There are all kinds of colors, textures, and products. Putting my makeup on in the morning is one of my favorite rituals for the day. Each morning I get to decide what kind of look I want to project and then use makeup as a prop to enhance that. What kind of goddess do you want to be today?

Foundation

If you are happy with your skin you probably don't want to wear foundation. If you are prone to acne or have an uneven skin tone, you may like to try foundation. I love mousse foundation because it is so light and protects your skin from the harmful effects of the sun.

Today many foundations serve dual purposes—to even out skin tone and provide SPF protection, or some have extra moisturizing properties and some have rejuvenating properties that help reduce wrinkles.

Choose a formula and a shade that gives you the kind of coverage you want. Liquids and mousse give the lightest effect. Sticks and creams provide more opaque coverage. You can also use a tinted moisturizer instead of a foundation.

Foundation spreads more easily on moisturized skin, so always moisturize your skin first. Even if you have very oily skin or acne, you still need a moisturizer. You can use a light jojoba oil to moisturize very oily or acne skin. Just a couple of drops applied to damp skin will work wonders.

Blush

Go easy on blush, as it is simple to overdo it. Use natural lighting to check your look. Gel blush is light, cream gives you more color, and powder blush gives the most intense color. Gel or creams work best for day, and cream or powders are good for evenings. Use blush sparingly—if you want more intensity, choose a richer color rather than applying a lot of a pale color. Swirl blush over the upper cheekbones and below the outer corner of the eyes. Don't go past the outer corner!

Eye Shadow

Remember the old saying "Blue eye shadow should be illegal"? Well, today anything goes with eye shadow. You can use blue eye shadow, red eye shadow, green eye shadow, silver eye shadow—there are no limits. Plus you can mix eye shadows to create your own colors and add glitter or sparkles to them for your own special effects. Don't mix too many colors together, though. Just as with paint, if you mix a lot of colors you will get a rather unflattering mud brown. Try layering colors—especially with a cream eye shadow—yellow over blue or apricot over pink. This gives a lovely shimmery effect. You can also add a dab of glitter to the inner corner of the eye or around the outer corner. Try sticking tiny body gems around your eyes, too, for an exotic look.

Lipstick

Never apply lipstick over the edge of your lips! I don't care how small your lips are, if you want a pouty look don't try that—you'll just look like a clown. Instead use a

strong color over your lips, then apply a dab of gold to the middle of your bottom lip. When choosing colors, try the color on your lips, none of this on the back of your hand stuff. The pigment is different there so it won't look the same on your lips. Get a Q-tip from the sales assistant and apply directly to your lips. Then go outside and check the color. Most department stores have harsh lighting and the color won't look the same once you are outside the shop. Many a time I have bought a lipstick color only to be disappointed when I got home because the color was a different tone or shade than what I thought I was buying.

Choose whatever lipstick colors appeal to you and in whatever texture you like best. I like different textures for different occasions. A bold matte lipstick looks good with a pale skin, pale eyes combo. Gloss looks good with strong eye shadow or for a healthy no-makeup makeup look.

Use a lip brush when applying lipstick, as it looks more professional. Plus the color will stay on longer.

With makeup and skin care products, more expensive does not necessarily mean better. Generally what you are paying for in the expensive lines is not quality but marketing and packaging. You can get just as good makeup from the drugstore as you can from high-end department stores. That said, however, if you have the money and want to splurge, go ahead. Sometimes you might find a color you like in the department store that you can't find in the drugstore—or vice versa.

Mascara

I love mascara—it makes your eyes look bigger. I think everyone should wear black mascara, no matter what their coloring! Of course most makeup books tell you to wear the shade nearest your natural coloring—light brown for blondes, brownish black for redheads. I say choose a color you feel great in. And have fun with colored mascara, too—like turquoise or blue or gold. I have been wearing crazy colored mascara for the last twenty years, ever since Christian Dior came out with gold mascara when I was a teen. I thought it was the most exciting makeup item I had ever owned! Now of course there are tons of wild colors. Bring out the inner rock star in you!

Makeup should be fun. Makeup should make you feel great. Makeup should not be something you feel you can't live without or something that you take too seriously. Think of yourself as an actress playing the parts in different roles and choose makeup that suits those roles.

To give your makeup a magical charge, place it near a window on the night of the full moon so the moonlight will charge it with magnetic properties. You can say a special prayer for the types of properties you wish your makeup to have.

Goddess Workout

Go through your makeup and throw away anything that is old, dried up, or you just don't love anymore. Then go to the drugstore and treat yourself to one great new makeup product.

Make an Altar for Beauty

If you have your own bathroom, you can do this in the bathroom. If not, use a corner of your dressing table. Make a special altar to Aphrodite and place objects of beauty on it. You can use silk scarves, lipstick, flowers, goddess figurines or pictures, perfume, pretty shells, glitter, candles—whatever comes to mind. In the middle of your altar put a photo of you that you like or a mirror to remind yourself that the divine Goddess of Beauty is now manifesting through you.

A Spell to Get Cute Boys to Kiss You

This is a spell I have used several times with great success!

Buy a candle in a pretty color that represents love to you. Pink is good for romantic love, red is good for passion, purple is good for a soul mate kind of love, and yellow is good for a happy, fun love.

374

On the candle, write the name of the person you want to kiss you. If you don't know who, just write *cute boy,* then write *kiss me, kiss me, kiss me.* Pray to the Goddess: "Dear Goddess, bring this boy or one even better to kiss me true before the next full moon." Burn the candle on the night of the full moon.

Once I did this spell and the guy I liked kissed me on the cheek a week later. Well, that was not quite passionate enough for me, so I did the spell again, specifying a juicy kiss. Two weeks later he kissed me with all the passion of an inflamed lover. It was quite an experience!

Aphrodite's Glamour

- Sparkly pink nail polish

- Any shade of pink clothing

- Her makeup is feminine, soft, and pretty

- Rose perfume

- Flower barrettes

Makeup

Put on a luminescent foundation. I like Revlon's "Skinlights." This will give your face a pearly glow. Use a sparkly blue eyeliner to define your eyes just around the edges of your eyelashes. The blue represents the sea from where Aphrodite came. Apply a pink cream eye shadow to your lower lids and in the crease.

Put lipstick in any shade of pink on your lips. Apply a dab of gold glitter to the middle of your lower lip.

For blush use a pink glitter gel and apply to the apple of your cheeks. You can also apply the gel to your collarbone and around your ankles for added glitz.

Clothing

Any shade of pink is great for Aphrodite—hot pink, pale pink, fuchsia. If you can't wear pink, then you can substitute red, gold, or purple.

Try:

- Pink sparkly jeans with a white T-shirt

- Little floral pink slip dress with silver clunky shoes

- Long pink skirt with a tiny tube top and golden slippers

- Accessorize with pink sparkly chokers or gold jewelry, rose perfume, and a large pink rose pinned to the corner of your skirt or on your T-shirt

Ceremony

Have a shower and get dressed in your pink outfit and apply your makeup. Dry your hair—loose is best for Aphrodite. You can add pink and clear crystal gems to your hair and flower petals, too.

Sit or stand in front of your mirror and light a pink candle. Play some music that is very soft and loving. Pray:

Blessed Aphrodite

Goddess of beauty, wisdom, and love

I know that you are the goddess of divine beauty

I know that you can make me a conduit of your beauty

Your wisdom and your love

Flow through me now

May your beauty be my beauty

May your love be my love

May your wisdom be my wisdom

I call upon the beauty of the universe to flow through me

Beauty of the stars, beauty of the sun, beauty of my inner holy spirit

Flow through me now

I invoke the holy spirit of beauty within me now

To radiate outwards to all who see me

All who hear me and all who know me

Feel the spirit of beauty illuminate you from within. Feel the energy build as a pink light within your heart area and spread outward throughout your body until it is emanating from every cell in your being. Reach upward and, using your imagination, draw beauty down from the stars, the sun, and the moon. Reach outwards and draw beauty in from the trees, the flowers, the air. Reach down and draw beauty up from the rocks, the rivers, and the earth. Feel this beauty of the universe weaving a magical gown of divine beauty all around you. When you are ready, look into the mirror and say: "Thou art beauty, goddess (your name)."

Aphrodite's Tasks for You

- Go out into the world as Aphrodite one day this week. How does it feel to be the Goddess of Beauty? Write down what you learn from your experience.

- For one week, throw away any negative thoughts you have about your appearance. As soon as they come to mind, say, "Thanks for sharing" and then think something wonderful about yourself.

- Every morning this week, look in the mirror and say, "Damn, I look fabulous!" Hey, it's your mind—you can think what you want. Practice saying it until you feel it. Say it as loudly as possible, the louder the better!

- Practice the walking beauty meditation each day this week. Draw in the beauty from all around you. Breathe it in deeply and feel it energizing your cells, beautifying you. Notice the beauty in others and in your life. Try to create beauty wherever you go through your thoughts, your words, and your deeds. Feel beauty come from deep within your heart.

- Read *The New Joy of Beauty* by Leslie Kenton—see Further Reading at the back of this book for details.

- Read *Moon Magic* by Dion Fortune (Weiser, 1979). This book is not about Aphrodite but it has some wonderful Aphrodite rituals in it. It also has a lot of great magical makeup information. It is written as a novel so read between the lines to get the magical knowledge. That will be good practice for you in "sorting the seeds"!

Conclusion

I hope you have enjoyed the journey through this book—I certainly enjoyed writing it. I encourage you to continue working with the Goddess on a daily basis. Start developing your own goddess glamours for other goddesses you would like to work with.

The best way to do this is to choose a goddess. Think about a goddess you would like to work with. There are many places where you can look if you are uncertain which goddess could best help you. You might like to look for a goddess within your own spiritual tradition, or perhaps you would like to work with a goddess from your ancestors' spiritual tradition. We all have "mixed blood" when it comes to our spiritual lineage. In my family, my father was Jewish, my mother was Anglican, and my grandparents were Maori, Russian, Scottish, and Irish. Each of those cultures has their own spiritual heritage. Write out your spiritual heritage. Make a family tree and go back a couple of generations. Find out what bloodlines you carry and what spiritual paths your ancestors followed. Choose the lineage that interests you the most, and then search for a goddess within that tradition.

Alternatively you can choose a goddess whom you have heard about but don't know very much about—you don't have to be related to her, per se. If you feel a special kinship with a particular faith or culture, then choose a goddess from there to work with.

Research Her Story

Once you have decided on a goddess, then begin to research her. Look for myths that tell her story. When you have found one myth, rewrite it as if she were telling the story, or from her perspective. Ask her to help you with this. Sometimes myths have a patriarchal veneer over them and if you use your spiritual senses to rewrite the myth, you may be surprised at how the Goddess wants her story to be told.

Before I begin to write I meditate for fifteen minutes. I lie down on my bed and imagine the goddess I will be writing about, and I start imagining her writing through me. I ask that she guide me and let me be a clear and accurate scribe for her thoughts. Then I play some instrumental music in the CD/ROM in my computer and type immediately into my word-processing program.

Find out what qualities the goddess is renowned for. Ask her for her opinion, too. One of the things I recently learned about the goddess Hecate that I didn't know before was that she has a wonderful sense of humor. She is a strong, powerful goddess who is often associated with death and endings, but she is also incredibly funny.

Create a Costume

What does the Goddess look like in any illustrations you can find of her? How is she described in myths or stories? What culture and time period is she from? How did people dress in those days? Use your intuition to guide you.

Putting together a goddess costume is fun. It doesn't have to be something that looks like a Halloween costume. It can be if you want it to, but it can also be more subtle than that. Like today, I am wearing a purple sparkly dress—one of my Moon Goddess dresses. Most people wouldn't know this is my Moon Goddess attire, they would probably think I was just wearing a purple dress. Today, however, I have important business to attend to, so I am asking the Moon Goddess for help in communication, clarity, and insight. I am also using purple because in biblical days purple was the color of royalty. I have been feeling a bit intimidated by the situation and wearing purple reminds me of my sovereignty as a Goddess Girl. I need to remind myself that I carry the divinity and power of the Goddess within me, and that I am a woman of power and can use my power wisely.

Create a Makeup Look

Again, use your intuition and what you know about the goddess you are working from and the culture from which she comes. Makeup is fun. Let it be an expression of your goddess self. With makeup you can create so many different faces for yourself. Today my makeup verges on the dramatic. I want to look powerful. I have a tendency to be too soft and accommodating sometimes. Today I need to stand up for my rights so I am wearing bold makeup—dark eyeliner, purple eye shadow, and dark fuchsia lipstick—to create a bold impression.

Use Jewelry, Perfume, and Accessories

These are the icing on the cake. If you are working with a moon goddess, use moon-based jewelry—either in jewels (pearls, moonstone, or silver) or in the shape of the jewelry (crescent moon pendants or triple moon rings).

Sometimes people like to have a special goddess ring that they wear on the index finger of their right hand. I had one for many years that had a female face on it in an art nouveau style. Start your own collection of goddess jewelry. You can find pretty pieces at New Age bookstores and at arts and crafts fairs. Also jewelry from your ethnic background or the ethnic background of a goddess you like is powerful to wear. I have several pieces of Maori jewelry and Celtic jewelry. Heirlooms are good goddess pieces. I wear my mother's jewelry when I want her protection or power to help me.

For perfume, wear what you like personally. I prefer essential oils to synthetic perfume because so many people have chemical sensitivities nowadays and synthetic perfume can give people adverse reactions. Go with the standards—rose for love, gardenia for intuition, sandalwood for sensuality. Let your own nose be a guide. Our senses are finely tuned so that whatever appeals to you will be the most powerful for you to use.

Invoke the Power of That Goddess

Always start with a shower or a bath before putting on your goddess clothes and, if possible, wash your hair. This is a purifying experience and it also helps you to clarify your intent before you get dressed, just as if you were dressing up for a special event. As you wash, imagine all the etheric debris you may have picked up during the day being cleansed off you.

Take your time to do your makeup and your hair. Think about the goddess you wish to invoke, talk to her while you put your makeup on, and ask her to help you. You might be inspired to try something new you hadn't thought of, or a particular product might seem to jump out at you from your cosmetic case.

Make sure your clothes are clean and freshly laundered. Then when you are ready, close your eyes, stand up straight with your feet gently apart, and hold your arms in the manner that seems most appropriate to the goddess you are working with. You will know what feels right; trust your intuition. Then think about the goddess you are invoking, think about what qualities she embodies, and see those qualities being embodied in you and flowing through your veins. Ask the Goddess to fill you with her love and energy. Ask for divine protection from any negative energy. Focus on the power of the Goddess and see her standing before you. Feel her energy merge with yours and pray to her from your heart.

Record Your Experiences in Your Goddess Journal

Write about your experiences of working with different goddesses in your goddess journal. This is your spiritual journey and a journal provides you with a map so you can see how far you have come, and it will give you guidance for the direction your life is yet to take. As you read back over the years, there will be events that you had forgotten, dreams that have come true, and heartaches that have healed. You will have your own goddess guidebook for how the Goddess has helped you, and this may be useful information for you to share with others. Not only that, but it will also be a beautiful gift to pass on to your own daughter or a special young person one day.

When I was a teenager one of my dreams was to write a book. I didn't know what kind of book at the time. When I was twelve I started writing a romance called *Love in Los Angeles*—I only got as far as the fourth page! Anyway, when I first started writing a goddess book, I knew absolutely nothing about writing books or how to get one published. It has all been a big learning curve for me. But I took classes, read books on writing and publishing, and kept persevering despite my own doubts and the setbacks and rejections I encountered along the way. Whatever your dream, the Goddess will help you to manifest it. You must put the work in and take action toward it.

If I can leave you with one final thought, it is: Please remember to use your goddess power every day. You have an unlimited supply of power at your fingertips. Use it. Practice using your goddess power every single day until it becomes automatic. Don't fall into the trap of playing the blame game and blaming circumstances, events, places, or other people for your misfortunes. I know it is really easy to do but it won't take you anywhere worth going if you do fall prey to blame or self-pity. Only you are responsible for making your dreams come true.

Remember the Goddess is all-powerful, all-knowing, and all-present. She can do great things. See her helping you every single day with whatever life hands you, and know that with divine power and divine love you can overcome any hurdle and accomplish great things.

May the Goddess guide you on your journey forward and may you see your own divinity each time you look in the mirror. Remember: You are the Goddess made manifest. Act like one!

With much love,

Catherine

Further Reading

Ashcroft-Nowicki, Dolores. *The Tree of Ecstacy*. London: Aquarian Press, 1991.

Austen, Hallie Iglehart. *The Heart of the Goddess*. Oakland: Wingbow Press, 1990.

Baring, Anne, and Jules Cashford. *The Myth of the Goddess*. London: Viking, 1991.

Barstow, Anne Llewellyn. *Witchcraze: A New History of the European Witch Hunts*. New York: HarperCollins, 1994.

Cabot, Laurie. *The Witch in Every Woman: Reawakening the Magical Nature of the Feminine to Heal, Protect, Create and Empower*. New York: Dell, 1997.

———. *Love Magic*. New York: Dell, 1992.

Caldecott, Moyra. *Women in Celtic Myth*. Rochester: Destiny Books, 1998. Eleven different myths of Celtic goddesses with accompanying interpretations.

Cameron, Julia. *The Artist's Way*. New York: Tarcher/Putnam, 1992. One of the best books ever written on practicing creativity and spirituality.

Choquette, Sonia. *The Psychic Pathway*. New York: Random House, 1994. A practical workbook for tuning in to your psychic senses.

———. *Your Heart's Desire*. New York: Random House, 1997. An easy-to-use workbook for manifesting your dreams.

Farrar, Janet, and Stewart Farrar. *The Witches' Goddess*. Custer: Phoenix Publishing, 1987. Includes a listing of over one thousand goddesses and a brief summary of each.

Graves, Robert. *The Larousse Encyclopedia of Mythology*. London: Reed, 1959, 1994, 1997.

Hay, Louise. *Empowering Women*. Carlsbad: Hay House, 1997.

———. *The Power Is Within You*. Carlsbad: Hay House, 1991.

———. *You Can Heal Your Life*. Carlsbad: Hay House, 1984.

Kanner, Catherine. *The Book of the Bath*. London: Balantine Books, 1986. Recipes for sixteen different baths including the moon bath, the love bath, and the twilight bath.

Kenton, Leslie. *The New Joy of Beauty*. London: Vermilion, 2000. I read this book when I was a teenager when it was first published and it is still the best book on beauty I have ever read. Excellent guide for inner and outer beauty.

———. *The New Ultrahealth*. London: Vermilion, 2000.

Llywelyn, Morgan. *Grania: She-King of the Irish Seas*. Ivy Books, 1987.

Mathews, John. *Celtic Warrior Chiefs*. Dorset: Firebird Books, 1988.

McCoy, Edain. *A Witches' Guide to Faery Folk*. St. Paul: Llewellyn, 1994.

Peale, Norman Vincent. *The Power of Positive Thinking for Young People*. London: Vermilion, 1998.

Pennick, Nigel, and Prudence Jones. *A History of Pagan Europe*. New York: Routledge, 1995.

Quant, Mary. *Quant On Make-Up*. London: Century Hutchinson Ltd, 1986. This fun cosmetic book has eighteen different makeup looks ranging from natural to wildly fantastic with detailed application instructions.

Ravenwolf, Silver. *Teen Witch*. St. Paul: Llewellyn, 1998.

Robbins, Anthony. *Get the Edge*. Robbins Research International, 2000. This audio program includes a cassette called Daily Magic that is worth the cost of the entire program.

————. *Notes from a Friend*. London: Simon and Schuster, 2001. A simple guide for taking control of your life.

Roberts, Nancy. *Breaking all the Rules: Feeling Good and Looking Great No Matter What Your Size*. London: Viking Press, 1987. The title says it all.

Ross, Anne. *Everyday Life of the Pagan Celts*. New York: Putnam, 1970.

Ross, Ruth. *Prospering Woman*. Novato: New World Library, 1995. A guide to creating prosperity in all areas of your life.

Van de Weyer, Robert. *Celtic Prayers*. Nashville: Abingdon Press, 1997.

Waldherr, Kris. *The Book of Goddesses*. Hillsboro: Beyond Words Publishing, 1995. Beautifully illustrated book of twenty-six different goddesses.

Wilkinson, Philip. *Illustrated Dictionary of Mythology: Heroes, Heroines, Gods, and Goddesses from Around the World*. London: Dorling Kindersley, 1998.

Index

Aborigines, 16, 57

accountability, 85

affirmations, 29, 32, 54, 64, 86, 221, 235, 370

Africa, 10, 17, 267, 270–271

Akashic records, 79

alcohol, 88–89, 182, 191, 317

allies, 10, 21, 23, 55, 108, 146–147, 264, 315

Amaterasu, 17

amulets, 8, 53, 131, 191, 205, 270–271

ancestors, 21, 28, 38, 44, 70, 128, 149, 190, 195, 202, 204, 245, 251–253, 256, 259–260, 262, 270–271, 350, 358, 379

Andraste, 12, 139, 141, 146, 149–150

angels, 5, 13, 23, 31–33, 55, 58, 60–61, 65–67, 71, 74, 83–85, 109, 128, 165, 192, 204, 215–216, 224, 259, 262, 283–285, 287, 295–296, 298, 331

anger, 58, 128, 133, 142, 149, 165, 214–217, 219–220, 243, 249–250, 254–257, 267, 297, 352

animate, 271, 297

Aphrodite, 5, 35, 46, 48, 50–51, 99–100, 258, 338, 361–377

aromatherapy, 26, 74

atheist, 24

aura, 24, 58, 62, 155, 165, 169, 296–299, 301, 319, 323

Aveda, 26

banish, 112, 189, 196, 198, 200–204, 336, 351

Baring, Anne, 10, 385

battle, 12, 46, 107, 119–124, 126–127, 134, 139–141, 145–149, 155, 218, 260, 264, 292, 305, 310, 321

beauty, 3, 5–7, 10, 17–18, 24, 31, 38–39, 41–42, 46–51, 53, 65–69, 71–74, 81–82, 91–92, 95, 100–101, 104, 116, 131, 146, 150, 154–155, 158, 173–175, 178, 182, 184, 187, 199, 210, 212, 225, 228, 241, 245, 252, 259, 261–263, 267–269, 274, 279–282, 284, 304, 307–308, 317, 326, 331–333, 338, 343–345, 349, 355, 361–363, 365–370, 373–377, 382, 386–387

bitterness, 16, 143, 179, 213–215, 217–219, 286, 327, 347

blame, 85, 108, 144, 213–215, 219–220, 259, 383

Boadicea. See Queen Boadicea.

boasting, 123, 127, 251, 260, 305

bodhisattva, 30, 213

body image, 331–334, 336, 342

Bonne Bell, 134

Brahma, 17, 173–174, 184

Bridget, 99, 157–171, 248, 290

Brighid, 12

broken heart, 158, 165, 183, 200, 309, 316, 349, 351–352

Browne, Sylvia, 197

Buddha, 24

Cameron, Julia, 40

Cashford, Jules, 10, 385

Celtic people, 5, 11–12, 15, 22, 45, 57, 67, 70, 90, 92, 119, 123–124, 127, 131–136, 139–141, 146, 149, 152–154, 157–159, 161–167, 169–170, 197, 248, 259–260, 264–265, 290, 303, 310–312, 315, 317, 352, 381, 385–387

ceremonies, 21, 30–31, 50, 52, 54, 67, 94, 96, 116, 133, 135, 154, 167, 170, 177, 179, 185–187, 202, 206, 225, 240, 263, 265, 271, 279, 282, 287, 290, 300, 322, 341, 357, 375

Chinese deities, 209

Christianity, 14–17, 22, 161, 287, 315

clairaudience, 56, 60, 232

claircognition, 56

clairsentience, 56, 62

clairvoyance, 56, 58, 68, 283, 297

Cleopatra, 100, 361

conflict, 145, 249

creativity, 8, 18, 21, 38, 40, 69, 72, 89, 94, 131, 146, 157, 173–174, 178, 183, 228, 231, 238, 272, 274, 291, 296, 320, 338, 348, 353, 385

Cronus, 327–328

crucifixion, 286

Cuchulain, 120–124, 127, 138

Day of the Dead, 189–192

daydream, 26

depression, 57–58, 125, 130, 133, 297, 357–358

diet, 13, 87, 325–326, 334–336, 339–340

Dionysus, 362

divine energy, 40, 47, 322

divine gifts, 106, 108, 113–115

divine life purpose, 109, 112

divine mind, 25, 27

divine wisdom, 37–39, 42, 79, 108, 117

DNA, 38, 195

Druid, Druidry, 17, 22, 25, 48, 160, 166

Earth Goddess, 15, 87, 95–96, 325–326, 328, 330, 333, 342

Earth Mother, 6, 15, 162, 307

Earth religion, 15, 17

Egypt, 11, 14, 131, 168

elder, 254

electricity, 28, 78

Emer, 120–121

emotions, 58, 60–62, 71, 81, 88, 95, 109, 125, 127, 139, 145, 213–215, 227, 231–232, 242, 252, 267–268, 272–277,

282, 293, 296–297, 305, 317, 319, 326, 350, 364, 366

empathy, 69, 86, 112, 114, 202, 222–223, 287, 355

energy drainers, 87

energy enhancers, 91

Enki, 103–108

Eridu, 104, 106–108

Eros, 362–363, 365

exercise, 61, 80, 85, 94, 125–126, 137–138, 168–169, 182, 185, 238, 250, 297, 301, 335–337, 340, 353

fairies, 5, 55, 58, 67–68, 100, 109, 165, 231, 298

fire, 11, 13, 16, 95–96, 150, 157–167, 170–171, 210, 243–250, 254, 256, 264, 267, 305, 313, 330

fitness, 124–125, 127, 273, 277

forgiveness, 61, 112, 209–210, 213–220, 223, 226, 353

Freya, 227–242

Gabriel, 284, 296, 300–301

Gae Bulga, 122, 124, 138

Gaia, 87, 99, 325–342

glamour, 99–101, 115, 132–135, 153, 169–171, 178, 185, 204, 224, 239, 262, 271, 281, 299, 301, 322, 341, 356, 374

God, 5, 11, 13–15, 17, 24–25, 33, 37, 46, 103–104, 106–108, 113, 124, 149, 159, 161, 164, 173, 176, 178–179, 190, 228–230, 247, 259, 269, 283–284, 286–289, 326, 328, 347, 362–363

Goddess, 3–21, 23–26, 30–75, 77–81, 83–96, 99–103, 108–111, 113–117, 119–120,

123–124, 128, 131–133, 136–139, 141, 144–148, 150–158, 161–162, 164–165, 167–171, 173–175, 177–191, 193, 197–204, 206, 209, 212, 214, 216–219, 221–222, 224–228, 230–231, 233, 235–236, 238–246, 248, 252–253, 255, 257–262, 264–265, 267–268, 272, 274–275, 279–284, 287, 289–290, 292–296, 299–301, 303, 309, 316, 318–321, 323, 325–326, 328, 330–334, 338–343, 347–353, 358–359, 361–362, 364–365, 367–370, 373–376, 379–383, 385

Goddess glamours, 99–102, 379

goddess of Laussel, 7

goddess of Willendorf, 7

Grania, 5, 45, 123, 303–324, 386

Grania Ni Mhaille, 45, 123, 313, 315

Greeks, 5, 12, 230, 311, 325, 327–328, 342, 362

grief, 195, 213, 215, 229, 285, 287, 317, 343, 346–348, 350, 352–353, 363

Haka, 136, 256

Hay, Louise, 26, 221, 386

Hecate, 290, 380

Hephaestus, 362

Hinduism, 16–17, 173

Huesuda, 189–207

Iceni, 12, 139–141, 315

inanimate, 271, 297

Inanna, 103–118, 338

India, 16–17, 100, 173–174, 178, 184–185, 209

inner goddess, 24, 37–75, 257–258

intentions, 25, 28, 31, 34–35, 107, 142, 155, 188, 202, 217

intuition, 40, 62–64, 69, 75, 109, 116–117, 220, 291, 364, 380–382

Japan, 17

Jasmine, 280, 300

Jesus, 30, 283–287, 289–290, 292, 296

jewelry, 50, 53, 66, 71, 84, 101, 116, 133, 135, 154, 163, 193, 225, 239, 262, 273, 281, 300, 356, 375, 381

Joseph, 284–285

Kabala, 21

Kai Karanga, 251–254

Kama Sutra, 178

Kenton, Leslie, vii, 91, 377

Krishna, 24

Kuan Yin, xiii, 17, 99, 209–226, 258, 338

La Llorona, 87, 343–359

Lady of the Lake, 290, 292

Lares, 13

law of cause and effect, 26–27, 215, 217

law of correspondence, 27

lorica, 149–151, 154–155, 219, 259–260, 262, 265

love goddess, 53, 179

magic, 3–4, 10, 16, 20–35, 39, 41, 43–46, 50–51, 53, 55, 57, 64, 66, 69–70, 77, 81, 84, 87, 92, 96, 100–101, 116, 122, 124, 131, 138, 146, 149–150, 153–154, 165, 169, 179, 185, 197–198, 202, 204, 230, 235, 238–239, 245, 252, 259–260, 265, 270, 272, 277, 290, 293, 295–296, 300–301, 306, 330, 333, 338, 347, 351–352, 357, 364, 370, 373, 376–377, 385, 387

magical toolbox, 29, 64

Mahuika, 16, 219, 243–265

makeup, 26, 49–50, 53, 101, 115–116, 133, 153–155, 169–170, 178, 182, 185–186, 204–205, 225, 239, 263, 280–281, 299–300, 322, 341, 356, 370, 372–375, 377, 381–382, 386

Maleus Malificarum, 15–16

mandala, 48–50

Maori, 16, 70, 131, 134, 136, 149, 244–245, 248, 250, 252, 256, 260, 263–265, 352, 379, 381

Marae, 245, 250–254

Mark Antony, 100, 361

Mary, xiii, 15, 17, 48, 99, 158–159, 164, 231, 258, 283–301, 386

Mary Magdalene, 286, 290

Mary of Bethany, 17, 290

Mary of the Celts, 158, 164

Maui, 244–248

meditation, 21, 30, 41, 48, 57, 64, 67, 71, 73–74, 83, 93, 165, 184, 187, 194, 216, 235, 250, 293, 332–333, 353, 357, 367–368, 377, 380

mehndi, 185

menstruation, 6, 289–290

mental fitness, 273

Mero, 211–213

Metis, 328

miracles, 22, 158–160, 167–168, 171, 277, 287

Moko, 131, 262–263

moods, 63, 95, 165, 228, 231, 272–275, 278–279, 282, 297, 313, 324, 327, 331

Moon Goddess, 16, 103, 283, 287, 292–293, 299–301, 380–381

Mount Olympus, 326

mythology, 12, 70, 90, 123, 157, 228, 248, 271–272, 325, 327–328, 386–387

myths, 4, 9, 230, 248, 303, 309, 362, 365–366, 380, 385

natural phenomena, 271

Neolithic Era, 9

New Mexico, 26, 48

New Zealand, 10, 16, 131, 244–245, 247, 260

Ninshubar, 107

omnipotent, 78

omnipresent, 79

omniscient, 39, 79

Ord Brighideach, 163

Oshun, xiii, 17, 267–282

overeating, 82, 87, 325–326, 334–335

ovulation, 290, 294–295

Pagan, 15, 190, 287–288, 386–387

Paleolithic Era, 6, 9

Penates, 13

perfume, 13, 48, 50–53, 101, 181, 185, 193, 240, 262, 270, 280–281, 300, 341–342, 374–375, 381

personal life purpose, 110–111

personality, 39, 43–46, 81, 110, 128, 313

physiology, 275

planetary life purpose, 110

power animals, 68, 204

prayers, 12, 21, 30–34, 41, 51, 53, 64, 74, 108–109, 115, 117, 137, 149, 154, 159, 161–163, 166, 168, 175, 177–179, 187, 190, 194, 198–203, 211, 213, 221, 226, 231, 235, 239, 256, 259, 281–282, 288–289, 300, 341, 369, 373, 387

priestess, 12–13, 25, 38, 66–67, 72–73, 105, 131, 179, 182, 186, 204, 216, 283, 289–290, 293, 301, 342

Psyche, 35, 362–365

psychic, 56, 68, 70, 72, 283, 291, 293, 295–296, 300–301, 385

psychic ability, 291, 295–296, 300

purifying, 96, 186, 214, 218, 240, 272, 382

quantum reality, 57

Queen Boadicea, 12, 99, 123, 139–156, 219, 259, 315

Queen Elizabeth I, 45, 123, 313

rage, 120–121, 141–142, 249, 254, 256, 352

religion, 14–15, 17, 22, 65, 209, 270–271, 287, 315

resentment, 213–215, 217, 219–221, 238, 297

Rio Grande, 343, 348

rituals, 31, 370, 377

Roman women, 311, 315

Rome, 13–14, 315

sacred heart meditation, 165

Saint Bridget, 157, 161, 168

sandalwood, 116, 185–186, 280, 300, 381

Sarasvati, 17, 173–188

Savitri, 175–177, 182

Scathach, 119–138, 150, 315, 338, 349

Selene, 290

self-responsibility, 85

sexuality, 66, 178, 180, 184, 187, 231

shaman, 25, 135, 240, 263, 270–271

Shintoism, 17

shrine, 13, 17, 47–48

soul, 73, 171, 176, 192–194, 212, 268, 270, 288, 292, 345, 347, 353, 355, 357–359, 367, 374

sovereignty, 69, 152, 154–155, 380

spells, 23, 30–31, 100, 154, 200–202, 259–260, 295–296, 374

spirit, 3, 7, 10, 24–25, 30, 38–39, 42–43, 46, 48, 60, 65, 68, 73, 87, 96, 109, 112–113, 128, 137, 139, 146, 175, 179, 181, 193–195, 197, 204, 206, 245, 252–253, 260, 271, 283–285, 287–288, 292, 297–298, 308, 357, 359, 361, 367, 369–370, 376

spiritual senses, 55–57, 59, 62, 73–74, 88, 251, 380

spiritual substance, 24, 29, 37–38, 57

spirituality, 24–25, 66, 69, 91, 178, 361, 385

Stone Age, 6, 28, 48

Summerland, 197

Sun God, 15

talismans, 131, 270

tantra, 178–180, 182

Tarot, 13, 49, 74, 108–109, 117, 177, 184, 272, 283, 293

tattoos, 51, 53, 119, 131–132, 135, 260, 262–263

Teweret, 11

tribe, 12, 25, 124, 126, 139–141, 244–246, 250–254, 263, 271, 315

underworld, 103–105, 209, 230, 328, 365

vampire people, 89

Venus, 7, 50

Vesta, 13

weapon, 122, 138, 149, 253

weight, 3, 20, 87–88, 119, 215, 329, 331, 335–336, 338, 340

Wicca, 22

wisdom, 3, 12, 17–18, 37–39, 42, 53, 69, 73, 79, 93–94, 103–104, 106–108, 116–117, 150, 177, 187, 196, 250, 261, 285, 290, 328, 349, 361–362, 375–376

Zeus, 327–328

Zulus, 271

Llewellyn publishes hundreds of books on your favorite subjects!
To get these exciting books, including the ones on the following pages,
check your local bookstore or order them directly from Llewellyn.

Order Online

Visit our website at www.llewellyn.com, select your books, and order them on our secure server.

Order by Phone

- Call toll-free within the U.S. at 1-877-NEW-WRLD (1-877-639-9753). Call toll-free within Canada at 1-866-NEW-WRLD (1-866-639-9753)
- We accept VISA, MasterCard, and American Express

Order by Mail

Send the full price of your order (MN residents add 7% sales tax) in U.S. funds, plus postage & handling to:

Llewellyn Worldwide
P.O. Box 64383, Dept. 0-7387-0392-3
St. Paul, MN 55164-0383, U.S.A.

Postage & Handling

STANDARD (U.S., MEXICO, & CANADA)

If your order is: up to $25.00, add $3.50; $25.01–$48.99, add $4.00; $49.00 and over, FREE STANDARD SHIPPING. (Continental U.S. orders ship UPS. AK, HI, PR, & P.O. boxes ship USPS 1st class. Mex. & Can. ship PMB.)

INTERNATIONAL ORDERS

Surface Mail: For orders of $20.00 or less, add $5 plus $1 per item ordered. For orders of $20.01 and over, add $6 plus $1 per item ordered.

Air Mail: **Books:** Postage & handling is equal to the total retail price of all books in the order. **Non-book items:** Add $5 for each item.

Orders are processed within 2 business days. Please allow for normal shipping time.
Postage and handling rates subject to change.

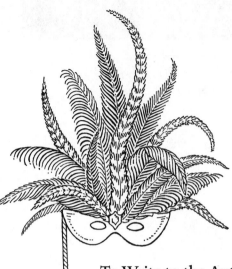

To Write to the Author

If you wish to contact the author or would like more information about this book, please write to the author in care of Llewellyn Worldwide and we will forward your request. The author and publisher appreciate hearing from you and learning of your enjoyment of this book and how it has helped you. Llewellyn Worldwide cannot guarantee that every letter written to the author can be answered, but all will be forwarded. Please write to:

Catherine Wishart
℅ Llewellyn Worldwide
P.O. Box 64383, Dept. 0-7387-0392-3
St. Paul, MN 55164-0383, U.S.A.

Please enclose a self-addressed stamped envelope for reply, or $1.00 to cover costs. If outside U.S.A., enclose international postal reply coupon.

Many of Llewellyn's authors have websites with additional information and resources. For more information, please visit our website at

http://www.llewellyn.com